ADVANCE PRAISE

"Allison Pelot has studied with me through the Chek Institute for many years. She's always been diligent with her studies, practices, and applications and is masterful in all aspects of holistic health — from performing comprehensive, holistic assessments of an individual's condition to creating holistic nutrition, exercise, diet, and lifestyle modifications that facilitate healing and personal, professional, and spiritual growth.

"Allison has been a popular guest on my podcast, and people always enjoy her depth of wisdom, creativity, and ability to 'think outside the box' regarding important issues of our day and ways we can all heal. Her book, Finally Thriving, is a true catalyst for positive change in the lives of all who read it and apply Allison's hard-earned wisdom."

—**Paul Chek**, Founder of The Chek Institute and
Holistic Health Practitioner

"Allison Pelot has a lot of magic to share. Whether it's getting better sleep, rebalancing some out-of-balance hormones, or how to deliver great podcasts, Allison has something valuable to say. And to make it even better, she is very humble and down-to-earth about all her knowledge.

"Allison and I were introduced through a close mutual friend, and we clicked. I've gotten to know her both personally and professionally and can tell you this for fact: Allison talks the talk AND totally walks the walk. It's part of the reason she is a great person to follow.

"Read this book. Enjoy this book. Implement the things that will help you in your life (you'll know which ones) and watch the magic happen."

—Mark England, Co-Founder and Head Coach of Enlifted

"From the moment I met Allison, there was something different about her: Allison's timeless wisdom and intimate knowledge of what it takes to help a person thrive is practical and free from any short-lived trends. She's helped me transform my relationship with food, and her work is what I recommend when someone asks me about the secret to my boundless energy.

"Finally Thriving is a lighthearted and masterful read   pick up a copy and allow Allison to open your eyes to just how easy it can be to feel your very best. I hope you'll love it as much as I do!"

—Hanna Bier, Freedom and Success Coach,
Energy Healer, Author

"A guide of relatable wisdom shared through the voice of your most trusted friend. With this book, you will experience valuable information presented in the most digestible ways. Allison speaks from the heart of her personal journey that really is all of our journeys. Enjoy tuning into those parts of you through her inspiring words."

—**Rosanne Grace**, Metaphysical Coach and Hypnosis Practitioner

"I have known Allison for years, and her ability to authentically transform herself is rare. Within the pages of her book, you will find her rare gift shared with you, the reader. Rare is the bird that not only rises early but also implements, ingests, and creates true change Allison is one of those birds. I would invite you to find yourself within the wisdom of her words and find your way back to finally thriving."

—**Jator Pierre**, Creator of HōL Method

"Few people have the passion or the drive to apply body, mind, and spirit to achieving excellence in their life. Those who do usually settle for excellence in one or two areas only.

"Allison Pelot began her journey toward self-mastery early in her life when she decided to pursue gymnastics. In the process of developing as a competitive athlete throughout her adolescence, she developed her mind and spirit along with her body so she could move beyond her fears and self-imposed limitations to consistently accomplish the seemingly impossible.

"Allison then went on to study and apply some of the most advanced practices for becoming fit on every level. Now she shares the secrets of her success with her private clients and the readers of this book as a holistic coach with expertise in tailoring exercise, nutrition, lifestyle, and a spiritual approach to living to fit people's individual needs and capacities. Finally Thriving is an enjoyable and informative guide to becoming who you always knew you were meant to be."

—Laurel Airica, Educational Entertainer, Communications Consultant, and Creator of WordMagic Global

FINALLY
THRIVING

FINALLY THRIVING

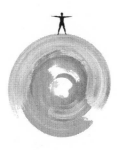

YOUR GUIDE TO EMPOWERED WELLNESS

ALLISON PELOT

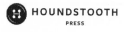

FINALLY THRIVING

Your Guide to Empowered Wellness

ISBN   978-1-5445-2586-0   *Paperback*

         978-1-5445-2587-7   *Ebook*

         978-1-5445-2588-4   *Audiobook*

CONTENTS

Dedicated to my dad,
who taught me that there really is life after death.

I was inspired to write this book on the day of my dad's funeral. It came in like a big download, and all of a sudden, I had so much I wanted to say. I never expected I'd be writing a book one day, but yet here we are.

My sister and I were with my dad when he passed, and we got to experience an incredibly sacred moment with him as he slipped away peacefully. I witnessed my dad's consciousness moving out of his body and into a different dimension of reality, and it was life changing.

I realized at that moment that there really is life after death. Death is not the end. Our energy is transformed in this life, and it moves on to experience something different in another life. It is important to learn how to take care of our bodies because they are what give us perspective and a frame of reference in this reality.

My dad always encouraged me to move toward what I was passionate about. He was one of my greatest supporters throughout my life, always cheering me on and showing up for me.

He was a talented musician, singer, and choral director. My dad had the ability to channel the energy of a group and direct their voices into sounding so harmonious. He even told me a story about how he got the football team to sing together one time (with no background in singing) and enter a choral competition—and they won.

He also had (and still has) a wonderful sense of humor.

My sister and I discovered one of his jokes written down on a piece of paper hidden under a bunch of other papers on his desk after he passed. We were stressing about whether to bury him or cremate him. Neither one of us could remember for sure what he wanted. Then we found this note...

"My only hope for a smoking hot body is to be cremated."

We both laughed out loud and felt his presence in that moment, remembering how he'd say...

"Don't take life so seriously."

INTRODUCTION

NATURALLY DESIGNED TO THRIVE

"My mission in life is not merely to survive, but to thrive; and to do so with some passion, some compassion, some humor, and some style."

—Maya Angelou

ARE YOU MERELY SURVIVING AND BARELY GETTING BY? OR are you doing fine physically but feeling unfulfilled mentally, emotionally, and spiritually? If the answer is yes to any part of these questions—and you're ready to upgrade your life significantly—then this book is for you.

Dr. Angelou was right. Surviving means having a reactive relationship to life. Things occur, and we just automatically react to them without a lot of reflection. On the other hand, when we thrive, we relate proactively within our lives. We choose what we

self-organizing

would like to experience, and then we create it. This is how we are designed to live and what will enable us to thrive.

It's actually more natural to thrive than merely to get by. Thriving is your natural state of being, yet we're inundated with medications, supplements, and life hacks that proclaim to be a solution to what comes naturally. The organs and systems of our body are self-maintaining—when we offer them the right fuel and enough exercise to operate optimally. Because our thoughts affect our feelings, which in turn affects our physiology, taking in the right nutrients and training the mind and the body pays high dividends.

The truth is, you came here already thriving, and you have all the answers within. My hope is that you realize the magnificence that is YOU: your true nature.

So, what if you learned to see the world—and your life—as half full instead of half empty, even amid the crises we are facing? Do you think you might have more energy to rise to the challenges in your life and more wisdom to face them effectively?

Is it possible to...

...*feel lucky all of the time?* yes

...*feel better at forty-five than you did at twenty-five?*

...*tap into your unlimited potential?* yes

...*feel grounded, calm, and anxiety-free?* yes

...create a body that you love living in?

...have abundant energy as you get older? yes

I say yes!

What's blocking you from this? There are more reasons than I can count as to why we never realize most of the things I've listed above. Unresolved trauma, negative stories and thought patterns, unconscious and unsupportive habits, mental health issues, or even just a feeling that "it's not possible."

It is my desire to share with you how I came to my own insights and turned my life around through my journey as a high-performance athlete, mother, energy healer, and holistic fitness and nutrition coach. To help you understand how the practice of creating a self-care ritual becomes magical because you learn how to take responsibility for yourself on all levels.

I've followed my passions, and they've led me exactly where I was meant to go every time. When I was five, I began a journey to learn about what my body was capable of. I started doing gymnastics in the backyard before I even took my first gymnastics lesson. Even at that age, I knew I wanted to see what this body could do. So, I began my journey by exploring physical movement as a gymnast and becoming a career athlete, competing from the time I was six to twenty-two years old.

Later in life, my curiosity led me to study almost everything under the sun related to the physical body and learn how to unwind the injuries I endured as a competitive gymnast. Because of all the physical therapy I went through at a young age, I became fascinated with my body's potential for regeneration and the process behind that.

After this, I dove deeply into the metaphysical and the relationship between the two. Over the years, I've had the honor and the pleasure of working with some of the most incredible teachers and mentors in the field of holistic health, nutrition, fitness, physical therapy, energy healing, metaphysics, and emotional wellness.

More specifically, my studies included holistic health practices, immune function, metabolic health, yoga practices, affirmations, goal setting, meditation for healing, Pranic healing, corrective exercise, abundance mindset, holistic nutrition, holistic lifestyle coaching, the mechanics of storytelling, inner child work, emotional life coaching, family constellations therapy, and so much more.

unique offering...

My experience in learning how to bridge the gap between the physical and subtle energetic body has led me to this point in my life, to understanding the physical body in a way that's allowed me to master my craft by working on myself and with thousands of clients, realizing there's still so much to learn, and approaching life with a childlike curiosity.

The subtle energy body as we see it in Qi Gong and reiki is something that's more real than we know, and acknowledging it as so is important. As is understanding the interplay between the two and navigating them in a way that will improve your life experience with synchronicity.

The word "humble" also comes to mind as I write this book. It drives me crazy when people follow experts more than they follow and trust themselves. As experts, we are taught to present as if we know everything, but this is often not genuine. Humility is not something you see too much of these days. It's what exposes our humanness to others, and it's how people connect with you on a human level. It's hard for most people to admit they don't know everything, yet we're either exposed to self-proclaimed experts or people who do not have enough confidence to commit to or stand up for an idea. Both come from a place of insecurity. I'm here to tell you there's a middle ground, and it's humility.

Being humble is authentic, and it's a way you can share your story and take expectations and perfectionism out of the mix. It's about giving other people the opportunity to come to their own conclusions and learn how to trust themselves.

To me, it means allowing—mastering your craft, which in reality is yourself, and then allowing what comes to come. If you make a mistake, do it with style, grace, and enthusiasm. Show others how you can shake it off, learn from it, move on, and keep going. This is a wonderful role model to set for others.

Showing your humility can even be a teaching moment for both yourself and others. You can make a joke out of it, and it can even lead to more creativity, laughter, and fun.

This book is also about admitting that I don't know everything, yet I have so much to share about what I've learned. This book is my gift to you, a guide to learning about yourself. And yes, while I believe I have very valuable advice and wisdom, it's ultimately up to you how you would like to use it. It's an opening to learn what you do not know and get curious about your life and the unknown aspects of it. My hope is that you'll use this book as a guide to discover and uncover parts of yourself in a way that brings you a greater sense of wholeness and joy in your life.

If there's one thing I've discovered, it's that you never get to a place where you know everything. Life would be pretty boring if that were the case, and even though most of us realize this, we don't actually live it.

I once met a woman in one of my emotional coaching intensives who was ninety-four. I couldn't believe that she still had the desire to work on herself at her age. At the time, I believed that I'd one day reach an age where I knew everything about myself and my work here would be done. I felt I could attain some kind of self-help completion, resulting in nirvana.

Little did I realize that's not the case, and at the age of ninety-four, there was more this woman wanted to learn about herself. It had never occurred to me until that moment that there's still room for learning about ourselves as we get older. I walked away inspired by her, realizing that our childlike curiosity never ends if we don't want it to. So why the rush to get to the finish line?

In this book, I want to share with you what I've learned and yet have some humility by admitting that I've made mistakes and have learned a great deal from them. I've also learned that it's less about knowing all the answers and more about sharing your unique perspective.

What I'd like for you to walk away with is a deeper sense of knowing yourself and what's true for you, inspired by a rekindled childlike curiosity for what life has to offer.

This exploration is dependent on two primary energies that infuse all of life: the physical and the energetic.

People talk about these two energies in many ways: polarity, yin and yang, masculine and feminine, receptive and penetrative. One of the most important things to become aware of is how these two energies interplay. The catch is if you identify too much with one or the other, you can get a bit lopsided or temporarily stuck. It's more about learning how to become the observer of your energy, direct it, and set clear intentions on how you'd like to live, thus harmonizing the two.

The physical and the energetic happen within all of us. But we can't always see aspects of our energy because much of it gets externally expressed in our world, so the illusion is that it's outside of us. We've also not really been taught the practicalities of the subtle energetic body and how to navigate this.

In this book, I'm going to share with you what I've learned about self-care, what it takes to truly love yourself and to tap into your unlimited potential, and why caring for ourselves and our bodies really just means learning how to love ourselves unconditionally. It's amazing when you realize that everything you need is in you. All you have to do is pay attention to it and learn to love it.

PART I

ALIGN YOUR MIND

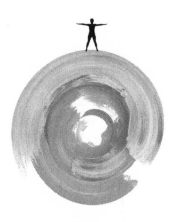

CHAPTER 1

WHAT'S YOUR DEFAULT?

"If you focus on the known, you get the known. If you focus on the unknown, you create possibility."

—Joe Dispenza

I'VE OFTEN WONDERED WHY THE COMMON NARRATIVE FOR MOST people is that the glass seems half empty instead of the glass being half full. Uhh...

Why do so many of us go straight to the worst-case scenario? Why isn't it a thing to go to the best-case scenario? Or, more directly: what we really want.

Part of it could be that we haven't yet defined what we truly desire. The other part of it could be that we've been conditioned to think this way by our parents, teachers, coaches, family, and friends. They weren't taught how to think optimistically either, and many of their stories have been passed down from generation to generation. No one questions it; most of us just continue this cycle of doom and gloom.

What is your default? Where does your mind go first?

I remember a time when I had certain beliefs, ideas, and stories that I'd ride or die with. Like I needed to dim myself to fit in or that I was a good person only if I sacrificed myself for others' benefits, therefore putting my own needs on the backburner.

In time, I came to realize that was not serving me, or anyone else for that matter. I was only hurting myself because I was not being honest with myself about what I truly wanted. I didn't yet realize that if I focused on the goodness in life, more would come, and I soon discovered a new way to be.

Your dominant perspective is everything, so pay close attention to it. Also, think about it: the likelihood of a situation turning out in your favor and for the good of all is just as possible as it not working out or going bad.

Both are possibilities. It really just comes down to what we want to create. Now that's a far stretch for some of us, especially if you've been identifying with your stories for some time now, but it doesn't have to be. We can simply change our perception and then watch our lives unfold into what we truly desire.

Let me introduce you to loving yourself, to optimism and positivity. This is how people who have been conditioned into limitation break out of that limitation and create something beautiful. This is where all of your creativity and innovation come from.

I'm not saying you should deny reality, which is different for everyone. But why not create a reality you want to live?

One of the most miraculous stories that comes to mind is that of Paris Robinson. I first met Paris when he was a guest on my podcast. He shared that he was shot four times in the chest, and he found himself paralyzed from the neck down. Paris couldn't feed himself, and he had to wear a diaper. The doctors would later tell him he'd need to be fed and taken care of for the rest of his life.

His defining low moment was when he was lying in bed one day and couldn't even swat a fly off of his face. Realizing he was powerless to even this small fly, he fell into an abyss of hopelessness and despair. Then he heard the voice of his mother (who had passed away) tell him that he must keep going and not give up. Hearing his mother's voice caught his attention, and so he thought about what he could do now to improve his condition. He had no idea where to start but then came up with an idea to visualize his muscle movement patterns in his mind while the physical therapist would move his arms for him. He also asked a nurse to put a sign on his door that said, "Please leave the negativity at the door." He no longer would allow any of the staff to talk negatively or focus on limits when they were in his room. Paris also requested that he start feeding himself as he began regaining more of his abilities in his upper body. He'd turn himself onto his stomach and do what he could to push himself up. It took a long time, but he eventually regained the use of his arms, and much to his surprise, he no longer had to wear a diaper and his sexual functions came back. This was all due to his focus and his change in perception. That's how powerful this can be. Paris realized his physical limitations in the moment and then did what he could do mentally to break out of what was perceived as limited. Paris knew he was the only person who could possibly know his own potential.

What can you control now? Start by letting go of the things you cannot control and focusing on what you truly can—like getting to bed on time, eating nutritious and delicious foods, getting sunlight, moving every day, and feeling grateful.

Begin talking to yourself with kind, loving words that describe more of what you want to create. Notice how much you use words like "shouldn't," "wouldn't," "couldn't," and "don't." Change these words out for phrases like "I get to," "I am," and "I want to." This puts you in a place of honesty and owning what you create rather than projecting what you don't want.

Set up a structure for yourself. This will create a sense of calm, trust, and confidence that is unshakeable. Yes, you may waiver at times or go off course, but we want the structure to serve as your new default, a routine you can always come back to when you notice you are out of alignment. This is what will ground you into your new reality.

If you don't know how to eat and move, hire someone to teach you those skills. Learn how to regulate your emotions; create some structure and framework around that which is unknown.

Learn how to create responsibility and accountability in your life by implementing these skills.

Believe it or not, you'll soon realize how this can open you up to infinite possibilities within your body, mind, and spirit. That's the kicker: you have to create a healthy foundation, and a healthy perspective is a key component of your foundation.

What would it take for your default to be love, optimism, and positivity?

I know it's easy to say, but you may ask, "How might I start?" You might think to yourself, *I want to be optimistic, but my old stories keep getting in the way.*

ACTION STEPS

We start by rewriting your story. Which is to say, imagine and then write your story how you'd like it to play out.

Action Step 1

First, open your imagination up to endless possibilities. For some, this is also the first challenge. Working with imagination can be extremely difficult for those of us who've stifled our dreams in hopes of fitting in and being accepted. In varying degrees, we limited the scope of our imagination because we learned somewhere that imagination and daydreaming were a waste of time.

7

Next, become aware of how easy or difficult it is for you to use your imagination. Then give yourself a free pass to daydream and see how it feels.

What comes up? Where does your mind go naturally? What does your "best life" look and feel like? Imagining the possibilities is paramount to begin moving toward what you want.

If it helps, imagine someone you see as a role model and then visualize yourself in their place. Begin training your brain to believe that you are fully capable of that.

I would use this technique when I was a gymnast. If I was afraid, had performance anxiety, or kept seeing myself fall, I'd rewire my brain to see it differently with this technique.

Action Step 2

Writing your story as if you're already living it and feeling it is also very powerful and brings the visualization into reality by grounding it. The written word is so powerful that it can literally change the course of your life through intention and focus. Saying it out loud (and even singing it) supercharges our words even more.

It can be something as simple as "I feel so good in my body right now" or "I love how I feel in my body." When we allow ourselves to visualize and *feel* our goals, we create the space for these experiences to emerge. This step is crucial for any lifestyle change or health habit you wish to integrate.

Second, think about what stories you currently hold and what they symbolize for you. Ask yourself, *Does this current story serve me? Did it serve me in the past? What parts can I keep, and what parts do I want to release?* Another way we can go about this is by getting curious about subconscious thoughts. Ask yourself, *Is this really true for me?* and *Where is this coming from?* If you need more support here, I recommend hiring a skilled coach or therapist who knows how to guide you through this process.

Action Step 3

Finally, write any limiting or unresolved stories you've been holding on to. Write this story out as if you were having a conversation and read it back to yourself slowly and with deep, low breaths between your sentences. Tune in to the feelings that come up and acknowledge them. On a scale of one to ten, notice the intensity of the feelings.

This process will help you integrate and resolve these stories. You'll soon realize that these stories no longer have the hold on you that they once did. Again, the process of letting go of your story can be incredibly healing, especially when witnessed and supported, so hiring a skilled coach or therapist is recommended.

The objective here is to uncover the subconscious thought processes currently running the show and to shift them as needed. By approaching this with curiosity, you bring a gentle awareness to that which is subconscious. It is the first step in carving out a brand new path.

Scientific Support

Ron Breazeale, "Thoughts, Neurotransmitters, Body-Mind Connection," Psychology Today, July 17, 2012, https://www.psychologytoday.com/us/blog/in-the-face-adversity/201207/thoughts-neurotransmitters-body-mind-connection.

CHAPTER 2

GET CLEAR
ON YOUR VALUES

OUR WORK EXAMINING THE STORIES WE TELL OURSELVES ABOUT our lives and who we are will help us in identifying what we value. When asked, someone might say they value things like "hard work, honesty, and sacrifice." There is nothing wrong with these things, but it's also likely that these values were "adopted" from the outside instead of cultivated from the inside. To take an inventory of what you value means identifying who and what is in charge of your life. This is the next necessary step in creating lasting, healthy lifestyle changes. Even the word honesty can take on a different meaning as it relates to that person's values.

For example, we often think we are being honest when really we're being loyal. Being loyal does not necessarily require respect, but instead calls for sacrifice. This can lead to resentment. The reflection here is that being honest with yourself is the value. The honesty you hold true to yourself will spill out to others, allowing each person to move forward in the relationship with respect instead of obligation.

Do you value what you were taught to value by your parents? Your family? Society? The media? Or do you perhaps hold values that are the exact opposite? Have you established your values from your authentic being? Or are they reactionary?

There are no right or wrong answers here; this is just an exploration. What are your values aside from what you learned from your parents and society? Are they different? Have you established them yet?

Here are some personal examples of my values:

- I value clean, organic, healthy food.

- I value feeling calm and healthy.

- I value time with my family.

- I value eight hours of sleep each night.

- I value a winding-down routine at night.

- I value a meditation session every day.

- I value movement every day.

- I value making the amount of money that feels good to me.

- I value my time outside and in nature.

- I value time with my clients.

- I value devoting time to myself every day.

- I value space for my own creative expression.

- I value love and support in my life.

- I value being around high-quality, loving people.

- I value time and space for cooking and eating three to four meals a day.

- I value and trust my body's innate healing ability.

- I value positivity, optimism, and joy.

- I value my self-worth.

- I value honesty with myself.

- I value integrity.

- I value making life fun, light, and easy.

It's okay if you haven't clearly defined these for yourself yet. Most people are unaware that their framework comes from outside sources and what they learned when they were young. Some letting go might be in order, and that's totally normal. The most important part is getting honest with yourself about what matters most to *you* as an individual. Then you'll see that you have a different value set within your family and a more diverse value set amongst your community.

Defining and owning your values is a way you can meet your own needs rather than looking outward to other people to meet those needs—especially in relationships. When we look externally to get our needs met, we become needy adults. When we can meet our own needs by becoming aware of how we can do this for ourselves, we can begin to parent ourselves. After all, your parents ideally were supposed to teach you how to become your own parent. While not all parents were great role models, hopefully most of us walked away with an idea of how we can continue to take care of ourselves by nourishing, affirming, and loving ourselves. If you didn't get that so much, not to worry; this book walks you through some ways you can begin to learn how to parent yourself.

There's a chance you may even still be rebelling against your parents' values instead of creating and discovering your own. This is equally as important to pay attention to. Many of us get mixed up in taking on the values of our family or community, and while there is nothing wrong with this, it can create a life that feels less fulfilling. The trick is to recognize what you're valuing, whether it's true for you, and then continually define and redefine what matters most to you. It will change over time as you grow as a person and experience more of life.

Once you have identified the basics, apply these values to what affects you on a day-to-day personal level. You'll begin to value your own opinion and what you truly believe about yourself instead of what others may be projecting onto you.

For example, I value a diet of healthy, organic food, but my parents don't exactly value the same thing—when they were growing up, everything was organic, so why buy something that's more expensive? In their eyes, it's a marketing scam, and from my perspective, it makes total sense to invest in organic food based on my life experience and what I know to be true.

Again, we get our first set of values from our parents, so it can feel almost like a betrayal to go against these values when we enter adulthood and redefine our own.

It takes courage to live authentically, by *your* values, and recognize that your values will change as you grow. But as you begin to work with values, you'll see how what you value builds the framework and foundation of your life. Your quality of sleep, quality of health, the kind of media you consume, how you treat others and the environment, how you treat your body, how you talk to yourself, how you spend your time, and the people you surround yourself with. Every single thing we do comes from a specific value.

Values play such a vital role in our evolution because without a clear awareness of them, you won't follow through. Goals won't be met if your values aren't aligned. You'll tolerate a lot of malarkey that'll take more energy, space, and time in your life.

For example, if I'm not aware of my level of value for a healthy body, I won't create the space for lasting change and awareness.

I won't have the wherewithal to make exercise a ritual or pass on processed, factory-farmed foods, and I'll never cultivate the level of energy that goes into creating a beautiful body. I won't make time for it.

Like by learning how to love my body, prioritizing movement each day, making time for a massage, taking time to cook and eat my meals, breathing with awareness, resting, learning a new self-care skill, learning how to eat and move, meditating, getting quiet, being present in my body, taking a walk, and the list goes on. Defining what the true embodiment of health and beauty looks like to me is key. Otherwise, I'm following what society tells me that looks and feels like.

Skipping this step will only create more work for you in the long run. All of the energy you spend, running around like a chicken with its head cut off—working to please other people, fit in, be accepted—is energy that you will send directly back to yourself by identifying what you value.

So why not reestablish that framework for yourself?

ACTION STEP

Write down five of your personal values and hang them up where you can see them.

Content Support

Paul Waters, "The Important Stuff—How Your Values Impact Your Health and Wellbeing," *Balance Health and Fitness Limited*, September 17, 2018, https://www.balancehealthand-fitness.co.uk/blog-page/2018/8/22/values-and-behaviour-change.

CHAPTER 3

IT ALL STARTS WITH FOCUS

"What you focus on will flourish."

—Anonymous

IF I HAD A DOLLAR FOR EVERY TIME I GOT DISTRACTED FROM my goal and was taken off course, I'd be a very rich woman. Like, we're talking millions. And while this is a natural part of being a human in the modern, digital world we live in, our distractions are a great way to examine what steals our focus.

Where do you focus most of your time and energy? Is it in what lights you up? Does it involve investing in yourself with self-development, joy, fun, love, and presence, or do you get swept up with the drama of the day? Are you busy distracting yourself *from* yourself, or are you creating space *for* yourself?

These are great questions.

Without a container, distraction becomes a form of self-sabotage. When it is conscious, distraction can be a nice break, time for play, or time for creative expression. The difference between the two is focus.

For example, I decided one day to turn my notifications off on my phone. I did this because I was tuning out, focusing on stuff I had no control over, and forgetting my purpose and my desires. I got sucked into a vortex of emotional chaos with nothing to contain it, essentially no context and no intention. No intention = no focus.

I'll be honest with you: I am the queen of distractions, and it is why many times I'm left feeling confused and disoriented after looking at a news blast or going down a rabbit hole on social media because there's no container for it. Truthfully, I'm just a curious person, and while I believe curiosity is a really good quality, the practice of focus asked me to get clear about where I'm directing that curious energy.

Regardless of how and why you get caught up in distractions, if there is no container for it, there's no focus, and your distractions become intrusive and detrimental. From my example, the phone notifications were literally stealing my focus and energy, making it impossible for me to accomplish the things that I wanted to be doing. Sometimes (actually most times), I completely forget what I was even doing in the first place, which leads to me beating myself up later for not being organized or present.

How many times has this happened to you? I imagine a sea of raised hands!

Just like our stories define our life and our values build the framework for it, where our attention goes is what flourishes. Once we decide what we need to get done in a day, staying focused on the task at hand is key. Whether it's a movement practice, health practice, spiritual practice, or business practice, a distraction, no matter how small or seemingly harmless, becomes a big problem if it consistently takes you away from your goals.

Do you want your phone, social media, or the news to decide what you do that day? Do you want Netflix to tell you what you prioritize, what you feel, and where you focus? I sure don't, and I bet you don't either.

Just like babies, kids, and plants need attention and focus to grow, so do your body, your creative projects, and all of your relationships. To love and appreciate with your focus is an act of doing.

ACTION STEPS

How can we begin to bring our focus into what matters most?

Action Step 1

Make mornings sacred: Let go of unnecessary distractions first thing in the morning. Mornings are sacred time spent with yourself. I get some of my best work done before everyone wakes up. I make it a habit not to get on social media until after I have my morning routine.

Allowing time and space in the morning for myself is essential. My morning routine is simple: sitting with my coffee and writing for thirty minutes. I meditate for ten to twenty minutes, and then I get ready for my day. I go for a walk and then move with my clients every day because I'm fortunate enough to have a job where I can do that. Then I make time for my family, perform my own movement practice, cook delicious meals, and get good sleep. Finding pleasure and joy in what I do are all what matter most to me.

Write down what you'd like your morning routine to look and feel like.

Action Step 2

Be selective with your calendar: I set time on my calendar for activities and skills I want to focus on and to grow. I check in with my soul every morning to find out what my soul wants to do that day. Then I write my overarching goals, purpose, and intention on a whiteboard and the steps to get there. I take a step each day toward my purpose with my focus and attention on those goals.

Take a look at your calendar. Is there anything that can be taken off? Is there anything that can be added? What would you like to be doing that speaks to your soul? What lights you up?

Action Step 3

Set social media boundaries: If you must get on social media, set some boundaries around it. Set certain times of day you'll log in and post, and by all means, take unnecessary notifications off your phone. Truly ask yourself if this notification serves you. If the answer is no, then get rid of it, pronto.

Set yourself up for success here by eliminating these unnecessary distractions.

Action Step 4

Post your values where you can see them: Go back to your values and go so far as to post them on your fridge. This makes it much easier to check in where you can see your values if you lose sight of them from time to time.

Some personal examples about how I want to spend my time and focus are that I want to spend quality time with my family, have an abundant life filled with fun, love, and joy, feel amazing in my body, have a business that is profitable, fun, and purposeful, and finally have time and energy to follow my own personal passions. If anything in my day doesn't bring me more of those things, I toss it.

The overarching purpose of my selected focus is my passion for teaching others how to find this within themselves. When I am telling myself positive stories about my life, I am better able to establish values that serve me, and from there, I can choose where I'd like to place my focus so that my positive experiences will continue to grow.

Lastly, it's important to bring love and appreciation in with your focus, especially as it relates to a person, relationship, animal, or living thing. Bringing us back to the idea that what you focus on flourishes.

CHAPTER 4

YOUR WORKOUT PERSPECTIVE

OUR PERSPECTIVE IS OUR TRUE POWER. EVERYTHING WE HAVE spoken about thus far really boils down to one thing: perspective.

For example, what if I told you you'd have a completely different outcome if you were to enjoy yourself and your body when you work out as opposed to just pushing through your workout like it's a chore?

If you focus on enjoying yourself while you work out, you're less likely to get injured and more likely to experience higher energy. This equates to choosing better things to eat throughout the day, getting better sleep, waking up rested... I think it's clear where I'm going with this. Perspective is everything, even in workouts.

In the past, I would sustain injuries that would literally put me down for weeks and months at a time. After a back injury that left me thinking I'd never walk again, I realized I never wanted to be in that situation again and that I must learn how to navigate my body better. What saved my back was learning how to *enjoy* my movement practice, not just get through it. I learned to slow down and get present with myself. That's not to say I don't work out really hard some days. I love how that feels too. But it's the awareness and appreciation of my body's limits and potential in that moment that are important.

I don't override my body's signals that I need to rest, slow down, or pay attention anymore. I honor my body's messages and learn how to decode what it is communicating to me.

I can almost hear you asking, "So I shouldn't push myself to work out if I don't want to?" This is where it gets tricky. We want our perspective while we're working out to be one of joy and presence, but how does this translate in those moments where we just *don't wanna*?

The difference is if you're enjoying your workouts and coming from a place of health, you're not getting that message all of the time. Feeling a lack of motivation can be a sign that you're not giving your body enough of what it needs in the form of nutrition and restoration. If you're sick or recovering from a physical ailment, you don't want to push through that, either.

ACTION STEPS

When it comes to your health: who are you doing it for? Often, we may not even be aware of this and are thinking, *Isn't this what I'm supposed to be doing?* While the answer to that question isn't "no," it doesn't feel very empowered, does it? Get clear on why you want a greater experience of health and write it out.

1. What messages are you getting from your body? You can only ignore yourself for so long before it demands your attention either through injury, energy slowdown, or illness. Are you unmotivated? Why? Are you having a hard time slowing down and instead pushing through? Why?

2. Are you enjoying your exercise routine? If not, what would you need more of to look forward to it? Start by moving toward activities and movements that you enjoy doing. I always first ask my clients what kind of activities are fun for them and what they'd like to work toward improving. Whether it's dance, sports, or even just walking, it matters. You can even ask yourself what you enjoyed most when you were a kid. This, many times, will lead you toward what your heart desires.

3. Finally, what personal beliefs do you have about both your body and yourself? For example, do you identify heavily with a past or present injury, or are you good at articulating your body's sensations? What are your beliefs about your body's potential? What are your beliefs about what you are truly capable of?

4. An example of this is that when I was younger, I got the idea that something was wrong with my body because I hadn't received the comfort I needed to feel supported. I had a ton of anxiety around changes in my body when I was younger, feeling like a hypochondriac at times. The hidden belief that something was wrong with my body wasn't true, yet until I became aware of it, this belief was driving my subconscious behavior.

27

5. Write down three or more beliefs you currently have about your body.

Scientific Support

Jory MacKay, "The Science of Staying Focused: It All Comes Down to a Weird Mix of Psychology, Habits, and Chewing Gum," Medium, February 13, 2017, https://medium.com/swlh/the-science-of-staying-focused-652bbc47df66.

CHAPTER 5

LEARNING HOW TO RECEIVE

CREATING A CALM DISPOSITION SETS THE STAGE FOR YOU TO receive what the world has to offer. When you're able to receive what the world has to offer, you automatically build trust that you will receive what you want in your life.

Why is this important?

You could say our ability to receive depends on what we learned from our parents, what we did or didn't get, and our level of trust that we'll be taken care of and in the universe's abundance. Many of us grew up in households that weren't perfectly nurturing, so our ability to receive was compromised. Receiving became something we needed to learn how to do on our own, and for some of us, we're still learning.

This can affect how much you prioritize yourself as well as the importance placed on recovery, rest, and your accomplishments.

If you are not allowing yourself to take in the goodness life has to offer by acknowledging your wins and receiving love from others, you will always be searching and never feel like you are doing enough.

Not knowing how to receive often translates to you searching outside of yourself to get your needs met. This inevitably leads to disappointment, resentment, and the continued feeling of being undernourished. The reality is, no one can meet our needs better or more consistently than ourselves.

You become a needy adult if you are always searching outside yourself to get your needs met. This inevitably spills over into your relationships.

The act of receiving really means allowing, but we have to feel safe and secure first. If your inner child does not feel safe, no one feels safe, so connecting again with your inner child and creating a safe environment from within is imperative. Learning how to receive is an act of nurturing yourself.

ACTION STEP

Connect with your inner child: Ask yourself: *What would five-year-old (insert any age that comes up for you) me have needed more of to feel safe? Loved? Nurtured? Whole? How would I have preferred to be parented? In moments of sadness, what did I wish I would have heard?*

If there is a specific memory, go with that and trust that this is what needs to be acknowledged within you. Imagine what that version of you looks like and see them in front of you. Ask them what they need. Once they tell you, talk to that younger version of yourself and tell them what you would have wanted to hear in that moment. When we can heal these parts of ourselves that are crying out for our attention and acknowledgment, we can begin to truly feel whole again by reconnecting with our inner child. Just acknowledging this within ourselves can be very powerful. Good job! You are learning how to parent yourself.

Content Support

Karen Mead, "Learning to Receive: 5 Steps to Opening Up," Tiny Buddha, accessed October 4, 2021, https://tinybuddha. com/blog/learning-to-receive-5-steps-to-opening-up.

CHAPTER 6

IT'S NOT PERSONAL

"Whatever happens around you, don't take it personally... Nothing other people do is because of you. It's because of themselves."

—Don Miguel Ruiz

ONE OF MY BIGGEST LESSONS IN LIFE IS LEARNING HOW NOT TO take things personally.

Spoken about extensively in Don Miguel Ruiz's *The Four Agreements*, not taking things personally is a massive cornerstone of a happy life.

Taking life personally is less about what others are doing or saying and more a reflection of unresolved issues within ourselves. The good news is that instances where we are taking things too personally are big opportunities for growth. They're showing us where our own attention is needed.

If something triggers you about what someone does or says to you, this is your first sign that parts of you are not in alignment with each other. Because when we are feeling conflicted inside, we start to see the conflicts outside of ourselves so that they can be resolved.

If, instead, you choose to play into the story of someone who did this to you, then it will perpetuate into something that blocks you from understanding yourself better. Hence never connecting to parts of yourself that desperately want to be heard.

When I reflect on this, I think about the times I'd give parts of myself away in exchange for loyalty from others. I was not prioritizing my obligations to myself and instead putting other people's needs first. When I'd give parts of myself away in exchange for loyalty from others. Later I realized when I took things personally from others, it was because I still had unresolved issues around my obligation to myself.

Putting my needs and values on the back burner was a huge sacrifice, and parts of me knew this. Taking things personally was a reminder that I was not honoring these precious parts of me.

Understanding this about yourself is really the most powerful move you can make. Searching inside for answers is a way that we can relieve ourselves from becoming a victim and ultimately take responsibility for ourselves in the best way possible. Then you can become the observer instead of the participant. Life begins to feel much lighter and easier, leaving you with a sense of calmness and confidence in your body.

The next time you feel yourself taking something personally, reflect on it.

ACTION STEPS

Reflect on a time when you were triggered by someone else. Why did that bother you? Is it really about you? What does that symbolize for you? What parts of you are conflicted?

Ask yourself, *Am I projecting, or am I reflecting?* The difference is that projecting takes the focus off of yourself and places it on blaming someone else. Reflection, however, is a wonderful alternative to projection because it allows you to become accountable and take responsibility for yourself in the best way possible. Reflecting opens up possibilities and puts you in a more problem-solving mode.

Get curious about what could be going on within you.

Scientific Support

Abigail Brenner, "How to Stop Taking Things Personally: Learning How to Hold Your Space and Keep Your Power," Psychology Today, August 26, 2014, https://www.psychologytoday.com/us/blog/in-flux/201408/how-stop-taking-things-personally.

CHAPTER 7

TRUST YOUR BODY (IT KNOWS WHAT TO DO)

YOUR BODY IS VERY INTUITIVE. AS A MATTER OF FACT, IT'S SO good at being intuitive it will continue to keep you safe without you even having to put any thought into it. It is a perfect system *of* systems that are complex and rely on each other to keep you alive and healthy. Your body doesn't even require you to fully understand how all of these systems work—just what supports it in its processes. It is *that* smart.

It is for this reason that when I see people over-intellectualizing nutrition and exercise, I know they are not experiencing true health. When we are in tune with the natural flow of our bodies, nutrition and exercise are simple.

For example, it took me a few years to realize I was putting way too much thought into eradicating candida in my own body. Candida is a harmful overgrowth of yeast that can manifest in a host of unfavorable symptoms in the body. At the time, I was under the impression that it could be eradicated. Counter to what I believed, I learned that candida not only can't be eliminated but shouldn't be. It's a part of you. If you got rid of candida, your immune system would shut down, and you would die.

The problem people run into with candida is that it becomes too dominant as a result of diets high in sugar and processed foods. Ironically, the fix for balancing this out was to teach my body how to digest good carbohydrates again and manage my blood sugar properly. You see, I'd been on a low-carb quest for almost three years back then. Sticking strictly to diets, like the antifungal diet, that don't allow any carbohydrates almost wiped my energy out completely, leaving me in a place of discontent wondering where to go next.

Luckily, I was able to get myself out of that low energy state by working with a coach who taught me that carbohydrates were good for balancing candida and for my body's energy systems in general. He explained that it's all about energy production and supporting the thyroid properly.

Since then, I've learned that we need the right kind of carbohydrates, like roots, fruits, and tubers, for carbon dioxide and thyroid hormone production. Mainly because carbon dioxide delivers and liberates oxygen and nutrients to our tissues, making it easier and more efficient to produce energy.

I'd found that the solution was to help my digestion move again and to support my metabolism by eating the right carbs at the right frequency, therefore supporting my body without over-thinking it.

This fundamental lack of trust that the body knows what to do is almost always what gets us into trouble. If we'd just give our bodies what they need, taking away excess and extremes without overthinking it, we'd naturally begin living a more vibrant life. This is not to say that when we're experiencing health problems we don't seek out professional help, opinions, and support. That is an essential piece. But remembering that our body is built to sustain helps us to work in concert with our bodies, not against them.

The trust we want to embody lies mostly in your body's healing process. You have an inner knowing that your body knows how to heal itself; all you have to do is give it what it needs. I think this is why the solution is always simple. If it were as complex as we make it today, we'd never have survived as a primitive species.

So why aren't we making it simple?

Because complexity *sells*. It sells you pharmaceuticals, it sells you complex diet protocols, and it sells you lots of supplements. In special circumstances, these things are needed. However, they are grossly overused and sold to us as an easy solution in exchange for giving our bodies real food, love, and support. We will clearly know when we truly need the intervention of prescription medication, an extreme diet, or an expensive supplement. But if these things become the go-to for every curious ailment: look deeper.

Allow yourself space and time to learn more and integrate the information your body is sharing with you. Physical healing takes time, and anyone who says otherwise is selling something. All that happens when we rush healing is more injury and pain.

Trust begins with awareness.

ACTION STEPS

Action Step 1

Body awareness meditation: Start by laying down on the floor. If you need something under your knees to support your back, go ahead and grab a pillow or bolster. I want you first to feel your body and the floor pushing back on your body. How does that feel? Are you feeling any areas that are tender or sore? Does it feel really good to let go?

Now, close your eyes and imagine a warm liquid light coming down through the crown of your head. Imagine this warm liquid light filling up your head, your ears, your nose, your jaw, and your throat. Notice any body sensations or emotions as you do this.

Now imagine this liquid light coming down to your shoulders, your arms, your hands, and then coming back to your chest, your heart, and your solar plexus. Fill these areas up with warm liquid light. Notice any body sensations or emotions as you do this.

Now bring this liquid light down to your abdomen, your hips, your buttocks, your pelvis, and fill these areas in with warm liquid light. Notice any body sensations or emotions as you do this.

Finally, bring this liquid light down through your legs, your knees, your feet, and your toes, and notice any body sensations or emotions as you do this.

Did you notice any areas that felt resistant, tender, or light? Write down which areas you felt blocked or any tenderness. Talk to any part of your body you feel needs the most attention and ask it what it wants to tell you and what it needs.

Write down what it says. Do your best to trust what comes to you initially and try not to second-guess the information that comes. We ultimately hold the answers; we just have to learn how to listen.

You can also build awareness by paying attention, observing, and learning when your body needs rest and regeneration. What are the signs? Are you exhausted? Are you over-adrenalizing and going into fight or flight mode? Your breathing will tell you what's happening. Are you breathing low and slow or fast and up high? Pay attention to how much activity you did that day or how much stress you've been under emotionally. Take that into consideration as you recover. Begin to pay attention to what is optimal for you in the way of food timing. Are you spreading your meals out enough throughout the day or taking in all your calories in one or two meals?

Support your body with the nutrients you may be deficient in. Notice how a blood sugar drop affects your mood, energy, and histamine response. If you supported your body this way, how would that feel, and what would that look like?

Trusting your body puts you in a relaxed mode, which is the most optimal healthy state. When your body is relaxed, you are better at recovering and healing. This also spills into having a more resilient immunity. On the other hand, a more stressed body will be more susceptible to illness and have a slower recovery rate.

Action Step 2

Journal: What did you discover during your meditation?

Did you need more food that day? Did you need more rest? Did you need more fruit? Was your body asking for less sugar, a break from alcohol, more sunshine? Did you need more movement? What kind of movement? Did you need more play?

When we come from a place of curiosity and wanting to learn more, and less of a place of fear, we're better able to build trust between ourselves and our bodies. This is the practice, and the practice builds trust and confidence.

Scientific Support

Rachel Hall, "The Body IS Intelligent," Unimed Living, accessed October 4, 2021, https://www.unimedliving.com/living-medicine/living-medicine/the-body-is-intelligent.html.

CHAPTER 8

ONE LOVE

"One love, one heart, let's get together and feel alright."

—Bob Marley

THE BLAME, SHAME, AND PROJECTIONS THAT YOU GENERATE and put out into the world come back to you.

This statement isn't coming from a karma perspective, though there is great merit to that. What I mean by this is that the way we perceive and define others is a reflection of how we actually feel about ourselves. Conversely, the degree to which you hold compassion for yourself is the degree to which you'll be able to hold and express compassion for another person. If you don't like parts of yourself, you're not going to like the parts of you that you see in other people either.

A simpler way of saying this is...

You are the practice.

I only know this because I've lived it, and it took me a long time to really lean into this one.

Devotion to self-love and self-care is truly a practice, especially considering it was neither modeled for us nor encouraged or taught. When we matter to ourselves first, the rest of life falls beautifully into place. Even, and especially, with our relationships.

Now you may think this sounds a little selfish, but I promise you it's not.

Arrogance and narcissism get confused with self-love, self-assurance, and confidence. The difference, though, is that arrogance occurs when we seek power from the outside. Instead of coming from the empowered place of self-love, arrogance and narcissism arise from an unconscious seat of self-loathing.

The confidence of self-love, on the other hand, is an expression of unconditional love for self. Think of someone in your life who exudes self-love. Their energy spills out onto others and uplifts the people and environment around them.

This concept is well-described by basic Buddhist principles in two of my favorite books by Von Galt, *Buddhist Principles of the Eightfold Path* and *Buddhist Guide to Manifest Parallel Realities*.

In *Buddhist Guide*, Galt describes what you're seeing as projections of issues you're dealing with from within, which are then seen as reflections of other people you come across as potential options and possible solutions.

For example, if you're having a particular problem in a relationship, you may come across other people who are having that same problem. You might see it as some reflections you don't like or some you do like. They may be a little further in the process, so you may notice how other people handle a parallel issue, and you might try that on for yourself.

This is so beautiful because it opens us up to a place of less judgment in what we're seeing in other people (which is really about ourselves) and into a place of more options and choices.

Think about it: how many times have you considered it acceptable to treat yourself poorly? I've done it. Let me count the ways...

I've discounted myself, criticized myself, invalidated my trauma, didn't prioritize or voice my own feelings, silenced my own voice, ignored my inner guidance, lost trust in myself altogether, and the list goes on.

We've all done this to some extent. But it doesn't have to be this way. Your internal dialogue is what shapes what you're experiencing about yourself right now.

In the movie *The Cosmic Giggle*, Mark England describes our internal dialogue like a vision board. He says no one puts anything on their vision board that they don't want, yet we tell ourselves what we don't want every day. It's the same thing; you are creating a vision board for your future with your internal dialogue. So why not talk to yourself with kindness and love?

Making "yourself" the practice helps you become aware of your habits, patterns, and projections. Once you're aware of these things, you can instantly begin to repair your relationship with yourself. How can you change your internal dialogue to something more loving moving toward more of what you want?

First, notice how you talk to yourself. If it's critical, tweak it a bit. For example, when I'd make a mistake in the past, I may have called myself stupid for doing that. What I tell myself now is, "Darn, I made a mistake. Everyone makes mistakes. I will remedy this the best I can." This is a more loving, supportive way of talking to yourself, and when you can begin showing yourself that level of compassion, it's so much easier to extend that out into the world to others.

ACTION STEP

Self-love begins with awareness and attention.

Begin by noticing the ways you talk to yourself.

Is it critical or encouraging? If it's critical, ask yourself why and explore where that could be coming from. Did you learn it from someone else?

When it's encouraging and supportive, how does that sound, and what are you saying? How can you bring that encouragement and support to other areas or activities in your life?

CHAPTER 9

USE YOUR IMAGINATION MUSCLE

"Imagination is more important than intelligence."

—Albert Einstein

MANY OF US NEVER REACH OUR FULL POTENTIAL BECAUSE IT'S not clearly realized in our minds first. We aren't using our imagination muscle enough, if at all. The truth is, our potential is a limitless concept. It costs us nothing to dream and visualize, yet so many of us shortchange this experience. We resist dreaming big because we run the risk of disappointment and failure.

Unfortunately, many of us, including myself, were taught that daydreaming was a waste of time. This limiting belief prevents us from stretching our imagination and exploring what is possible as we get older.

Using my imagination muscle allowed me to tune in to what I truly wanted to create.

Imagining what you'd love in your life and how you'd like to feel is key to creating the life you want. More specifically, imagining a body that feels amazing is the first step in attaining a body that feels amazing. Imagination teaches you what is possible; it reveals to you what you truly want. If we don't allow ourselves to dream, we miss out on possibilities, new ideas, and opportunities.

Albert Einstein also said, "Creativity is intelligence having fun."

In the realm of creating a greater experience of health and vitality, it is necessary. If you can't imagine what perfect physical health would look and feel like, you won't be able to maintain the determination and fortitude that is required on the path to get there.

When you tap into your imagination, you start getting naturally curious about your process. This sparks your inner creativity, which is ultimately what makes the process fun. If it wasn't fun, we probably wouldn't hang in there for very long. Hence why so many people get super motivated to get in shape every January and then quickly fall off the wagon within weeks of starting. It's because we've never been taught how to go outside the box and imagine something greater. Align your mind with what you'd like to do first. This takes imagination.

ACTION STEPS

Action Step 1

Build a vision board: My go-to for this is to create an old-fashioned vision board. I know, it seems "cringey," as my teen would say, but it works, and it's so much fun.

If you don't feel artsy and you want to make it easy, I suggest going straight to Pinterest and creating a vision board there. This will help you better bring your vision to fruition, and let me tell you, for those of us who struggle to dream big, this is a great way to give yourself support until you build up that imagination muscle.

If you are an artistic type, go all out. Head to the art store for a canvas, buy magazines you love that feature the themes of what you're working toward, and get markers, glitter, paint, stickers, and anything else that speaks to you.

Acknowledging your inner desires and wants is a big deal.

As a somewhat grounded and realistic person, I realized I wasn't giving myself enough space to expand my imagination, therefore not allowing myself to play.

I limited myself to a certain level of success that was somewhat controlled for fear that I would not get what I wanted, so why bother dreaming about it. Keep it simple, I thought.

Action Step 2

Visualization meditation: Another way I was able to strengthen my imagination muscle was through visualization in meditation. I used this method often when I was a gymnast. I'd start by visualizing my favorite Olympic gymnast doing the skill I was working on over and over again until I could visualize myself in her place. This worked great because I'd more times than not be able to translate that into executing the skill I was preparing my mind for.

You see, gymnastics is very much a mental exercise. We used to have this saying, "You're psyching yourself out." That means even though you've practiced this move a million times and you know you have it, you're thinking too much about what could go wrong with it. I'd avoid psyching myself out by using visualization meditation. I would spend a few moments visualizing myself performing the moves I knew perfectly. You can do this too with your health and with activities you'd like to do. You can even use a visualization meditation for post-injury, imagining how it would feel when you are fully healed and doing all the things you'd like to do.

Connecting to the light meditation: An important aspect of this that I learned and use with my clients is to first connect to the light. This puts you in a place of energetic alignment during your visualization meditation.

You can execute this meditation by connecting to the light through the top of your head and slowly bringing it down through each energy center, or Chakra, and to all parts of your body until you get to your feet. Imagine this as a waterfall of light or a liquid light coming into each part and crevice of your body, clearing out that which is no longer serving you and filling you in with love, abundance, and opportunity.

Then imagine a cord coming down through the bottom of your feet and to the center of the earth and connecting to a crystal. Trust that whatever color comes to mind at that moment is the color of the crystal. Imagine the crystal sending loving light back up through the cord and radiating up through your body. This is grounding you into this subtle energy expansion.

Then imagine the light coming from below and the light coming from above, both merging in the area of your solar plexus. Imagine this light then radiating out like a bubble expanding out past your body, filling it in with pure love and light. Then expand that bubble out past the building you're in, past the city you're in, past the country you're in, and then out past the planet. You can even expand this light out past any planets you're connected to.

Now that you're connected to the light and grounded in your body, you can visualize your future self. What do you look like? What are you doing? What feeling do you get when you see yourself? Do you have anything to share with yourself? As you get familiar with yourself and feel complete, thank yourself and then watch yourself disappear.

Write these insights down and save them to reflect on later.

This is important because the energy you are living now is what manifests your life in the future. So connecting with your future self is important to see and feel so that you can begin to take ownership of what you are creating now.

Action Step 3

Journal: How was the experience of building your vision board? Were you surprised by what you created? Did you feel anything open or soften within you as you worked?

What shifts did you find during the visualization meditation? Did you discover anything new or experience new insights? Keep track of what you find in these meditations and watch for signs that they're beginning to manifest in your life.

Scientific Support

Shaunacy Ferro, "How Imagination Works," *Popular Science*, September 16, 2013, https://www.popsci.com/science/article/2013-09/how-imagination-works.

CHAPTER 10

OVERCOMING THE FEAR OF CHANGE

CHANGE IS UNCOMFORTABLE. JUST LIKE WITHIN SOMEONE'S spiritual journey, in the area of health and wellness, we come across dogma, politics, and industry beliefs that are heavily ingrained in our consciousness.

There have been moments in my life when my entire foundation of reality in my own health journey has been blown to pieces because I uncovered another circle of truth that I was not aware of previously. Now, in the second half of my life, I've become pretty open to that process, but at first, it turned my world upside down.

It's become somewhat acceptable to shame people for having another school of thought. Even getting curious or questioning a reality they've grown up in can be risky.

Could it be cognitive dissonance, or do we lack the skills to look deeper and broaden our perspective about what's possible? I think it could be both.

Cognitive dissonance occurs when a person holds contradictory beliefs, ideas, or values and is typically experienced as psychological stress when they participate in an action that goes against one or more of those. This idea originated from Leon Festinger, an American social psychologist.[1]

When a person receives new information that doesn't seem congruent with what they've learned, they'll fight the new information to make some kind of sense as to why that information exists and then dismiss it while going back to their more familiar thoughts and beliefs. It's when you literally have separation within the parts of yourself.

In this situation, most people are left feeling a deep need to prove and defend their beliefs because they're simply not taught how to make peace with the separation within themselves.

The truth is, all beliefs are malleable. Beliefs could even be regarded as opinions; they come and go and don't feel as permanent as a belief. So if that's true, then why are we feeling such a need to prove and defend?

In my experience, this reflects a deep fear of change. As humans, we are here to grow and learn. With that goes changing and letting go of beliefs that we've outgrown because we've discovered a larger circle of truth. This is our natural process.

It's when we are in conflict with parts of ourselves that we feel the need to prove and defend. For example, you may have developed

---

1 "Cognitive Dissonance," Wikipedia, last modified September 20, 2021, https://en.wikipedia.org/wiki/Cognitive_dissonance.

or are currently developing a new value that may be different from what your parents taught you or what society is telling you.

If you lack the awareness around what is happening here, you may come across someone who represents that part of yourself who wants to change and create a new value. This might trigger you if you're not aware of this dynamic.

Pushing this away or denying this process within yourself will stifle your growth. I think it's important to define cognitive dissonance within ourselves because it's rare for us to be aware this is even going on.

It's totally normal for your ego to want to keep you safe, so any information or ideas that are scary to you or create a catalyst for change are understandably going to shake things up. What's not normal is the long-term distress we create with separation within ourselves, dismissing parts of ourselves by wanting to hold on to old beliefs in the name of being right and feeling safe.

When your need to grow is greater than what you know.

This happens as it relates to how we see our bodies and our energy. You can see how we can find resistance within our own bodies because we have separation from within. If you wish to change your body, you have to also check in with any cognitive dissonance within yourself. Because remember, anything that you're experiencing outside of yourself, you're also experiencing inside because it's a reflection and an opportunity to grow.

The question is, what is real to you? What is your truth? I can tell you it's always evolving, changing, and expanding. It's a practice in itself to learn how to perceive this way.

How do we find peace with cognitive dissonance? We start by the practice of becoming open to the nuance of ideas and your own perception. You also start with being open and willing to change your beliefs. As I mentioned earlier, if we can think of our beliefs more as opinions, they don't seem so permanent. We don't get so attached to our beliefs and see them more as a reflection of what we think we know in that moment.

True power is finding yourself in other people and letting other people find themself in you. This is the power of "oneness." Becoming whole again. After all, it's an illusion that there's any separation at all.

Can you practice saying, "Let's agree to disagree" if you don't agree with someone? This shows you have respect for another person's perception and also allows you to hold space for your own growth.

ACTION STEP

Ask yourself these questions, and feel into the answers.

Write the answers down or just acknowledge them to yourself.

1. Where is there conflict within you?

2. What are you resisting that is begging to change?

CHAPTER 11

GROUND YOUR MIND BY TUNING INTO YOUR BODY

YOUR BODY IS ALWAYS SPEAKING TO YOU. LEARNING HOW TO understand your body's language is one of the most important skills you'll ever use. Your life depends on this for you to feel healthier, stronger, and more energetic, resilient, and vibrant.

As a young gymnast, I learned how to overcome pain. Chronic pain from the constant impact of landings and lots of pain from injuries like torn knee ligaments, broken ankles, feet, and toes, and four surgeries and a stress fracture in my lower back.

I learned how to overcome both physical and emotional pain so well in fact that over the years, I became resilient to it. Mainly because I had to if I was going to make it as a gymnast. A very logical side effect of this was learning to override my body's natural signals of needing rest and recovery. It laid the foundation for some of my greatest physical challenges as I got older.

As I got older, I started experiencing severe digestive distress, low energy, and a low sense of self-worth. Because I had trained my body for so long to "go hard," I'd find myself severely depleted after moderate workouts—needing one to two full days of complete rest to build my energy back up again. By the time my second child was born, life had become unmanageable because my body was severely nutrient-depleted.

I had to learn to tune in to my body in ways that I never had before. Learning how to articulate my body's sensations was also helpful.

You can probably guess it's been my lesson in life to learn how to allow, surrender, and be. Many of us find ourselves here. It's probably been the most challenging thing for me to acknowledge within myself, but by seeing the value in slowing down, I soon realized how magical life can be.

Learning how to manage your energy flow and listen to your body is key to your success.

Since then, I've seen so many of my clients go through this on many levels, finding themselves in a place of not being able to do the activities they used to because they didn't have the energy to do it. They're no longer able to push through because they've used those reserves already, and pushing through was all they knew. By the time they get to me, they're at their wit's end. After seeing countless functional medicine doctors and practitioners, they are left feeling like they've tried everything and nothing is working.

I always say if it feels too complicated, you're probably making it too complicated. Very rarely do we look at the obvious when it comes to our health. It's all about your lifestyle. What part of your life are you perpetuating that isn't working for you anymore?

So many people override this feeling of needing a change in their life, hoping that a magic supplement protocol, a restrictive nutrition plan, or even medication will fix everything and allow them to continue on with the current lifestyle they are living. In other words, "a quick fix so I can keep doing what I've been doing."

What if it's really about your lifestyle? Be honest with yourself and ask, *Is my lifestyle serving me? Am I running around like a chicken with my head cut off, never getting to enjoy the fruits of my labor, or am I allowing time for what I'm passionate about, for the people and experiences I love? Am I prioritizing myself, or am I putting myself on the back burner?*

What if it's about the lack of interest and time we put into ourselves? We may naturally gravitate to do the ten-minute abs or *Buns of Steel* workout in the hope of somehow unintentionally creating that body.

Ask yourself...

Is ten minutes a day enough time to give to yourself? Are you enjoying the time you are giving to yourself?

Now, I'm not shaming anyone for wanting to do those kinds of programs; just do them consciously. I know how appealing it can sound to be able to knock something out that quickly that most of us put off on a daily basis, and I realize that most people don't really want to put the time and the effort into learning how to become an exercise guru. I get it, but my question is, why not explore why you're putting yourself off if that's the case?

Why can't you give yourself an hour a day? Whether it's a walk or a combination of a walk and a meditation, a run, or a check-in with a proper warm-up stretch and then a nice enjoyable workout. Something you enjoy doing. Why not explore that? Do you even know what you enjoy?

Begin by tuning into how your body feels when you move. Are you checking in, or are you checking out?

Being present in your body is a great start. I always do my best to keep my clients in their bodies when they work with me. I'm constantly asking them how that feels and where they feel that movement when we're in a session together. I want them to learn how to be in their bodies. This way, they are better able to embody the feeling of strength, stability, and confidence.

It's a common thing for many of us to check out of our bodies. An easy way to learn how to stay in your body is to check in with more awareness and take the monkey mind out of the movement.

HOW TO CHECK IN
WITH MOVEMENT

I help my clients with this by repeating key movement sequences that provide a daily check-in for them to connect with their bodies. They walk away learning more about their body and address what needs attention in the moment.

When we're sequencing movement, we're also taking the monkey mind out of the movement. You can't drift off into thought when you have to focus on contralateral movements. For some people, it's like chewing gum, standing on one leg with your eyes closed, and patting your head. In other words, it takes a lot of concentration.

This is necessary because it provides a framework for you to build on. Get the chattering mind out of it so that you can learn how to listen to your body. Your body will always reveal what's going on; you just have to know how to listen.

We also work on letting feelings and emotions move through the body during a movement session. The feeling of stability, strength, and balance are important to connect to in your workout because connecting to what you feel in your body will change your perception and, soon, your external reality.

You have the power to change your entire experience of yourself this way. Plus, you'll feel better, and people who feel better will naturally attract the goodness life has to offer. You'll also be available to give life your best because you have the energy to do so.

Another way I recommend tuning into your body is through your breathing. If you ever feel like your thoughts are circling over and over again, leaving you feeling anxious and exhausted, connect to your breathing. Slow down the rate of your breath and bring the breath down into your diaphragm and belly.

Switching your focus to your breath is one of the best tools I use to get me back into feeling in my body again. When we get caught up in our thoughts, we also tend to get caught up in our stories. When we get swept away by our stories, we're no longer able to be in the now. We're either in the past or the future. Being in the now is all we have, really. Eckhart Tolle made the concept of being in the now popular with his book *The Power of Now*.

It sounds like a wonderful notion, but do we really know how to implement being in the now? The best way I've found to do this is by first examining our stories. You know, those stories that subconsciously run your life. You may not be aware of them, but they are there, and they are tricky. When we're able to release these stories by breathing them in, they lose their hold over our lives. It becomes less of an issue and even sometimes comical.

Even more powerful is writing your story out, slowing down your rate of voicing it, and adding in a breath between sentences. This will change the way you feel about your story forever. It's powerful, and it puts you back in the present moment.

Another technique I teach my clients is how to begin a nose breathing practice at rest or during light exercise. This automatically gets you into your parasympathetic nervous system, rest and digest, and gets you out of flight or fight.

ACTION STEPS

Action Step 1

Sound healing: Sound healing with your own voice is a great way to ground your body and quiet your mind if you have a hard time getting still and meditating. You can connect the sound to toning each energy center or Chakra in the body too. There are so many ways we can develop this wellness relationship with our bodies. A simple way I love to use sound healing is through vocal toning. In Stewart Pearce's book, *The Alchemy of Voice*, he describes how you can heal yourself by toning with some key vowel sounds, which are:

- Root Chakra sound: LAW

- Sacral Chakra sound: VOM

- Solar Plexus Chakra sound: RA

- Heart Chakra sound: YOM

- Throat Chakra sound: HA

- Third Eye Chakra sound: OM

- Crown Chakra sound: KEY or HE

I recommend repeating each one three times before moving on to the next one.

This is a wonderful way to both clear your Chakras and put you into a parasympathetic mode by activating the vagus nerve.

Action Step 2

Take yourself on a wellness date: These are all things you can do on your wellness date. I suggest going on a wellness date with yourself every day. A wellness date is time spent with yourself, giving your body that time and attention it craves by doing something you enjoy.

It can be any of, but not limited to, the following:

- A vocal toning session

- Listening to a recorded crystal bowl session while lying on the floor

- Your favorite guided meditation

- Walking in nature absorbing the goodness

- A ten-minute stretch session

- Dry brushing your body

- Self-massage, especially around scars

- Silicone cupping

- A trip to the farmers' market

- Preparing and eating a new delicious, nutritious meal (something you haven't made before)

- Eating on the floor, like a picnic or in your backyard

- Eating by candlelight either outside or inside

- Taking an Epsom salt bath

- Doing yoga

- Taking the time to enjoy your workout

- A physical activity you enjoy like riding your bike or roller skating

- Dancing spontaneously or having an impromptu dance party

- A sauna session

- Foam rolling your whole body

- A bike ride

A wellness date includes anything that allows you to give your body the love and attention it deserves. Just like a child, a plant, an animal, or a relationship, if you ignore them or criticize them, they will not thrive. Getting into a ritual of making yourself a priority will let your body know how much you appreciate it.

I love to walk in nature, sit in the sauna, or use vocal toning as tools for learning how to spend time with myself. What do you enjoy? How can you take your body on a wellness date? What does your body crave?

Content Support

Alanis Morissette, "How This Singer-Songwriter Tunes Into Her Body," *Mind Body Green*, last modified September 3, 2020, https://www.mindbodygreen.com/0-23541/how-to-tune-in-to-your-body.html.

Scientific Support

Linda Graham, "How Tuning In to Your Body Can Make You More Resilient," *Greater Good Magazine*, October 3, 2018, https://greatergood.berkeley.edu/article/item/how_tuning_in_to_your_body_can_make_you_more_resilient.

CHAPTER 12

YOUR EMOTIONS AND YOUR PHYSIOLOGY

DID YOU KNOW THAT YOUR EMOTIONAL BODY IS A HIGHLY INTELLIGENT feedback system? It guides us toward the things that bring us joy and expand us, and they alert us when we are treading into areas that are unsupportive, painful, or dangerous. We typically view our emotions as uncontrollable, random, maybe even chaotic, but they are actually very precise and can be worked with in practical and powerful ways.

From a wellness perspective, emotions are a tool your body will use to tell you things are out of balance, physiologically. However, many of us haven't learned that our emotions and body are connected, so we rarely put it together that feelings of sadness, irritability, or frustration could be *physical*.

Feelings of emotional pain, anger, and moodiness are all related to fatigue, for example.

A slow metabolism can result in restlessness and anxiety. An underactive thyroid can give rise to insomnia, memory loss, and episodes of panic.

In fact, depression has been newly linked to an imbalance of the microbiome in our intestinal tract.

In Dr. Broda Barnes's book, *Hypo-thyroidism: The Unsuspected Illness,* he talks about how low thyroid function affects your emotions and mental health. Again, because we haven't been taught to connect our emotions to our physiology, these things go unnoticed, resulting in the breadth of chronic illness that so many experience in these modern times.

It's fascinating to me because what this means is that true health is way easier and more attainable than we make it. We just have to pay attention. Our emotions can be our beacon, signaling to us what is out of balance before we reach a point of no return. We can start to do this by examining what nutrients we could be deficient in and balancing our blood sugar properly.

Most of us are familiar with the term "hangry": the feeling of hunger and anger at the same time due to low blood sugar. It is a cute, slang term for hypoglycemia. It's something that doctors used to look at and consider heavily when it came to the state of one's health. I've definitely experienced this firsthand growing up and witnessing how my parents responded to waiting too long to eat.

If there's one thing I know about my family history, it's that hypo-glycemia is real. If only I wouldn't wait five hours to eat, I might be a different person, and I know this because balancing blood sugar is the cure.

What I know about myself is that I'm no good if I skip a meal. Believe me, I've tried every diet known to man, and it's circled me right back to the notion that I have to prepare my meals and eat fairly frequently. At the very least, I need three square meals a day.

My friend Josh Rubin of East West Healing described this beautifully in his analogy. Would you hold off on feeding your infant if they were crying and obviously needing food? Would you say: "Let me wait until tonight to feed them and ignore their incessant crying, hunger, and need for attention?"

Of course you wouldn't. But this is what we're doing to our bodies when we ignore our physiology's consistent need for fuel in the form of food. I've learned over the years that I need to regulate my blood sugar by having at least three square meals a day for my body to be in balance. Otherwise, my mood drops, and I become irritable and self-critical.

If this goes on long enough, I notice there's a breakdown in my connective tissue, and I start to get inflamed. I'm less flexible, both mentally and physically, and my quality of life begins to diminish—all from skipping a meal!

How can you begin to get to know your blood sugar balance better? Everyone is different, so here are some things to pay attention to and journal on.

ACTION STEP

Over the course of a week, pay attention to any emotions that arise within you and when. What is happening when you're feeling this? How does your body feel? Have you eaten? If so, what did you eat? How does your stomach feel? Write this down.

Conduct a thorough observation of your emotions and moods and how they relate to your body.

Here's an example of an entry:

> This afternoon, I felt a drop of energy and a rise in irritability. I realized I hadn't eaten in almost five hours. My stomach was rumbling, I had a low-grade headache, and my breath was shallow. After eating lunch, I felt myself begin to balance. My headache went away, and I felt energetic.

At the end of the week, look for any patterns. It may be as simple as needing to adjust your meal schedule, but if there is a consistent pattern of unease, it may be time to seek professional or naturopathic help.

CHAPTER 13

HONOR YOUR PERSPECTIVE

"If experience is the best teacher, there's nothing that comes close to the experience of life."

—Michael A. Singer

THERE'S VARIATION WITHIN WHAT YOU'RE FEELING AND EXPE-riencing, and it's always different than what someone else may perceive or experience. Much like putting too much weight on another person's perspective, we also miss the nuance and depth within our own reality.

My reality can be different than yours, and that's okay.

This both gives me a sense of possibility and inspiration and helps me not get too attached to the feeling. What if we could love ourselves for who we are and know our worth? What would the world be like then?

Knowing there's variation gives me a sense of permission to be myself and find humor in life despite what's going on around me. Not getting stuck in my emotions but instead allowing them to move through.

How can we learn how to value the process instead of only focusing on the results? How come some people say that we must ground ourselves in reality and stop dreaming or kidding ourselves that we have any control over the universe?

Others might say to have faith, and the universe will provide. If you plant a tomato seed, you have some sense of faith that if you water it and give it good soil and sun, it'll grow into a bigger plant and give you tomatoes.

I think there's nuance in this. The key isn't to attach to any particular dogma; it's to find out what's true for you. How do you do this? You learn how to play.

It really doesn't matter what you think reality is—what matters is whether it's working for you. You'll come across a ton of people in your life that are truly confident they have the answer.

This is because when we put so much weight on what other people perceive and share, we are not considering that what we have experienced in our own lives is very different from someone else's.

I say this because rarely do we realize this when we make ourselves wrong and another person right. You have a unique experience and perspective, and another person has theirs. Realizing this liberates us from second-guessing our experiences because there is no right or wrong, just choices.

While it's great to appreciate other people's opinions, you also have to decide for yourself based on your experience of what is true for you regardless of what anyone else thinks. Now that's bold.

I got to the point where I was grounded so much in my "so-called" reality that I'd totally lost touch with my ability to imagine possibilities and opportunities that I desired. I did this because it felt safe and stood a very low risk of disappointing me.

The problem was that I had unmet desires that I was not acknowledging. I wasn't being honest with myself about what I wanted, and so I was denying myself an opportunity to manifest those desires.

I let myself off the hook by taking no responsibility when it came to the energy I brought into every situation. I also noticed I wasn't acknowledging my childlike curiosity, and my inner child made sure to let me know.

This was me. I didn't realize the magic in life happens through play. Yes, as an adult, I had to learn how to play. I had to learn how to make mistakes and not beat myself up about it too. I had to learn how not to take life so personally. I had to learn how to stop making up worst-case scenario stories about how I experienced other people.

But first, I had to tap into my own imagination and acknowledge my desires. If I wanted to believe that the universe provides, I'd believe the universe provides because it works for me. I do things because they work for me. I've put principles into practice. I don't do them because of someone else's belief about themself that they've projected onto me.

I'd put myself and my needs on the back burner long ago, and my inner child was ready to let this go and play again. To become the unrealized artist I always wanted to be.

You see, I chose to be an athlete long ago, all in the name of meeting what I thought were other people's expectations of me. I desired to be both an athlete and an artist.

I chose an athlete, and boy, oh boy, did I sabotage myself in so many ways because of it. My inner child was not happy with this decision, so I was left feeling like I needed to combat what I felt others needed or wanted of me by sabotaging the situation so that I couldn't be seen as that shining light I was born to be.

I remember feeling like there was so much pressure on me to perform. I felt it physically, and I felt it energetically by feeling closed in and stifled all of the time. I had sacrificed my playful artist for a serious athlete.

It left no room to be me. My deep desire as a kid was that all I ever wanted was to do it for me, not for anyone else. The issue when we work out, eat, or perform for other people is it stifles our inner child and doesn't allow us to play, make mistakes, or find joy in the moment.

This also requires you to look at your own judgment both about yourself and other people. If you're judging other people critically, you're most likely critically judging yourself too.

I remember being most judgmental of myself because I was resisting what I truly desired, all in the name of meeting other people's expectations of me. Then it all backfired. My parents got divorced. I realized I'd wasted all of this time trying to please other people and keep the family together, and so I rebelled hard. As a teen, I was pissed.

At the time, I didn't understand how meeting other's expectations while putting my own desires on the back burner could be a sacrifice of parts of me that were precious. I didn't know how to be discerning, only judgmental. I wasn't able to tell the difference between critical judgment of self and others and the use of discernment.

Now with that being said, judgment is natural for everyone. It's impossible to go through life without any judgment. We're in physical bodies, and we need judgment to be able to apply discernment in our lives to people we want to be around and situations we want to take part in.

Only judgment can get to a place of criticism and loathing if we're not careful. Watch this within yourself and pay attention to where that judgment is coming from. Is it coming from a parent, society, a friend, or yourself? If it's healthy judgment, you'll know the difference; that's called discernment.

If it's unhealthy, you can bet your bottom dollar you'll probably feel pretty bad or even self-righteous afterward. Tune in to the feeling the judgment reveals. This is the nuance I'm talking about. Our many levels of reality and how we all experience ourselves is what we want to put our energy into, along with the ability to judge our situation well.

ACTION STEP

List one to two desires, and then write this sentence:

I am the highest self-expression of me, and I...

Fill in the blank with a phrase that describes how you'd like to feel and experience life when your desires are met as if they already are.

Here are some examples:

I am the highest self-expression of me and...

- I have poise and grace.

- I have confidence.

- I love the ocean.

- I am smiling.

- I am laughing.

- I am captivating.

- I am magnetic.

- I uplift the entire room.

- I am telling my story, and it's clear and captivating.

- I am helping millions of people understand themselves and live a joyful life.

- I am happy and joyful.

- I laugh all the time.

- I am my true expression.

- I am expressing myself all out, not holding back.

You can apply this writing exercise to anything you'd like to experience in your life. This will help you to embody the feeling that is associated with what you'd like to create.

If you want to take it one step further, write these every day for a week.

This will put you in a deep connection with what you desire.

PART II

CONNECT TO
YOUR BODY

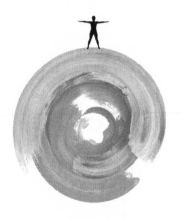

CHAPTER 14

ARE YOU WORKING *IN* OR WORKING *OUT*?

THERE IS A DIFFERENCE BETWEEN A "WORK-IN" AND A "WORK-out." I learned this lesson years ago from one of my teachers, Paul Chek. He coined the phrase "working in," which was influenced by ancient movement practices like Qi Gong, as well as more modern movement modalities such as Feldenkrais. The difference between "working in" and "working out" is that "working out" is an outward expression of your energy, and "working in" is a building up of your life force energy.

What these ancient movement practices all have in common is that they're tools for calming the nervous system so that you go into a deep healing and highly aware state. They also create awareness around your energy flow and release energy blocks in the body by moving them through.

These movements give you an opportunity to not only feel into your body, but also to regenerate your body by tapping into your natural energy source—sometimes known as life force energy or chi. Both "working out" and "working in" are equally valuable, but working out tends to be a more common concept for most people. The truth is, we need balance in both of these areas, which is why when we're deficient in either of these, we feel out of balance.

What does it mean to work in? The best example is Qi Gong, a specific movement practice that moves energy through and re-energizes the Chakras, or energy centers in the body. The idea behind this practice is that the slower you move, the more life force energy you can create and build in your body.

Although Qi Gong is an ancient spiritual movement practice, you can apply this concept of slow movement to any movement you do. You can walk very slowly with a walking meditation. You can do a hip lift or a squat very slowly and repetitively. You'll get a similar effect. Your nervous system will calm down, and your body will then have access to deep rest and recovery. The slow movement moves you into your parasympathetic nervous system, which is your rest and digest mode.

This goes for your breathing too. Tuning into your breath by bringing it slow and low and slowing your movement down will aid the body in regeneration. You can easily learn how to integrate "working in" movement into your weekly practice. Your body may even feel tingly, or you may feel a surge of energy come up. Some people have a big yawn and feel the need to take a nap. Whatever you feel, it's your body's unique way of letting go of excess stress and tuning in.

This is so valuable to connect to because when you can begin to feel your body's expression of release and energy flow, you can tap into your body's innate healing potential. It's everything because when I say healing, I don't just mean healing a wound or getting over a sickness or disease. We're always healing or regenerating our physical bodies. It's important to understand if you're working out regularly. Knowing when to rest and knowing when to move is crucial for creating a healthy, vibrant body.

ACTION STEP

Hip lift:

Lay on the floor on your back, bend your knees and rest your feet into the floor. As slowly as possible, begin to lift your hips off of the floor until you reach the top. Make sure you are pressing with your feet and heels to lift your hips. Then as slowly as you can, release your hips back down into the ground and imagine your hips melting into the floor. Repeat this meditative movement for at least ten repetitions.

Feel the energy come into the pelvic and hip area. You may feel tingling or a sensation of energy or chi coming into this area of your body. Move with your breath.

Find more "work in" exercises available at www.finallythriving-book.com.

CHAPTER 15

START A RECOVERY PRACTICE

THE ONLY DIFFERENCE BETWEEN A YOUTHFUL BODY AND AN older body is the rate of recovery, healing, and regeneration. The factors involved vary largely, but without a strong basis of regeneration, this process can diminish over time.

When I learned this, it was a serious game-changer. I realized that if you have the tools and skills to recover, you can create quick regeneration and a more youthful look and body over time. For example, when you go through periods of stress or strain, your body will move through those states more quickly, integrating and releasing that tension instead of holding it and storing it. You'll instead be able to train your body how to regenerate and heal consistently.

Having enough energy reserves in the form of food is also important in your recovery process.

This understanding is gold. It opens up the gate for a long and sustainable youthful life, no matter how old you are.

The key is both replenishing the energy you've used and knowing how to regulate your energy.

A proper plan of recovery can include but is not limited to eating delicious, high-quality food, balancing blood sugar, massage, self-massage, skin-rolling, nose breathing, hot tub soaks, acupuncture, sauna, stretching, resting, walking, active recovery, foam rolling, cupping, healthy sun exposure, light therapy, going to bed early, and getting enough sleep. Just to name a few.

Good digestion can be added to the list and is essential because a slow digestive system leads to waste getting stuck and putrefying in the gut. This leads to a host of unseen stresses on your body, namely a sluggish liver and detox system. Not only does it lead to poor health in general, but it also takes up so much energy.

Poor digestion can lead to low energy, fungal infections, parasites, hormonal dysregulation, candida overgrowth, and autoimmune issues. A healthy, functioning digestive system does not allow for any of these issues. A fired-up digestive system is meant to work like a furnace for these kinds of unwanted bugs, growth, and inflammation.

When you have more energy from a healthy digestive system and more digestive motility, you'll have the energy needed to recover, which in turn nurtures healthy hormones and helps you detox more efficiently.

Another key factor in recovery is circulation. If you can create better blood flow in an area that had restrictions, it's going to heal so much faster. There are many techniques for this, but walking on a regular basis is a great way to get started. Another favorite method of mine is foam rolling. It helps to better circulate blood around muscle and fascia, especially if I have a compacted or restricted area I'm having a hard time getting to by stretching. And of course, massage is excellent too. Whether it's self-massage, acupuncture, cupping, or seeing a massage therapist, this is a practice that is both therapeutic and deeply relaxing.

You can also use infrared light therapy to regenerate cells, heat via a sauna to support your thyroid, or aid sore muscles via an Epsom salt bath.

Many times, our lymph nodes need a little extra help because of the sedentary lifestyle so many of us have adapted to. Rarely do we learn the tools of recovery and how these are essentially tools of circulation.

You create circulation through movement, and if you can't move without restriction, you work on lifting the restriction through stretching, fascia release, and increasing mobility. Mobility, in some respects, is all about training your body how to move the way you were born to move. Connect to your unique movement signature.

This goes the same for energy in the body. When we have restrictions in the fascia, this creates an electromagnetic energy block.

Therefore if you can create more circulation and free that area up, you can have energy flowing freely up the chain.

This supports a higher level of both performance and vibrancy.

Honestly, I love all of my recovery tools and strategies. I do my best to integrate as much recovery time as I can. I've no doubt felt a difference in my own energy (way more at forty-eight than in my thirties). I feel better and have been able to keep a youthful look. I have a high quality of life and feel like I have the freedom and energy to move the way I want to. It gives me a sense of grounding and empowerment when it comes to my body.

I also find this to be true in the clients I work with, all because they've learned how to repair their bodies and create a regular recovery practice. It's a skill we all could benefit from.

Stretching can be a key component of a recovery practice too. I recommend trying different key stretches and learning where your tight spots are. Generally speaking, these are areas you'll most likely need to come back to time and time again.

I tell my clients it's okay if they have to keep coming back to these areas. You'll probably never reach a place where it'll be totally resolved, but it'll get so much better, and you'll begin to train areas in your body to stay open and move better overall simply because having a lifestyle of sitting mostly during the day will require a regular practice of unwinding.

You'll also increase your range of motion in a joint just by stretching and rolling. Dynamic stretching is my favorite kind of stretching because it's a way you can begin to train your body how to move into its natural end range and push that a bit in a safe way.

Dynamic stretching is a type of stretch where you are moving through, not holding. It's a great tool to use before your workout because it stretches and activates your stability muscles, while passive stretching—holding your stretch for sixty seconds or longer—before a workout can sometimes shut off stability muscles. That's why I recommend passive stretching at the end of your workout or before you go to bed.

Of course, stretching can also be helpful in bringing circulation to an area too. Stretching before you go to bed and even lying on the floor can help to reset your body and spine, aiding a deeper, more comfortable night of sleep.

ACTION STEP

Lying on the floor at the end of the day has also been very good for getting me back in my body and feeling grounded. It's also a great opportunity to surrender to not having to do anything. I just lie there and feel my body.

Lying on the floor gives me an opportunity to feel any pushback in my body. Try this yourself. Lie on the floor and feel where there are any discrepancies. Does it feel good? Does it feel uncomfortable? What part of your body needs your attention?

CHAPTER 16

THE MANY BENEFITS OF NOSE BREATHING

NOSE BREATHING IS ONE OF THE EASIEST WAYS TO A HEALTHIER metabolism, better digestion, a higher oxygen uptake, and a calmer disposition. It sounds almost too good to be true, but when you understand the basic principles behind nose breathing, it totally makes sense—and it's magical.

I first discovered the magic of nose breathing when I read Patrick McKeown's book, *The Oxygen Advantage.* He talks about how most people are mouth breathers the majority of the day and how this unhealthy habit can even change our metabolism. Surprisingly, many athletes are even prone to it.

This blew my mind. I'm always excited to learn that something as simple as repatterning our breathing could lead to more energy, better digestion, a higher recovery rate, and better sleep. How easy is that? When a person predominately mouth breathes throughout the day, this puts them mostly into sympathetic nervous system mode, our flight or fight response.

If we're in this mode most of the day, our body stays in a constant stressed state, and our metabolism becomes less efficient. We also lose the ability to retain enough carbon dioxide, which carries and liberates the oxygen to the tissues.

This decreases our oxygen uptake, lowering our threshold to deliver oxygen to tissues, thus making it harder to exercise efficiently. We make it harder on our bodies by increasing the workload.

The more CO_2 production you have, the less muscle soreness you'll experience after a workout. This is an easy fix. By training yourself to breathe through your nose 90 percent of the time, you can reduce your lactic acid response by retaining more CO_2 in the body, thus lessening your inflammatory response after your workout. This makes recovery much easier and your motivation to work out again way more accessible.

What's more is that if we're not breathing through the nose, we lose out on our body's natural ability to filter the air we breathe through our nose. Air wasn't really meant to come in and out through the mouth; that's why we have nose hairs. This improves your immunity and your immune response exponentially.

Your body knows what to do; you just have to learn how to support it.

What's also really cool is that we can affect our disposition and perspective by repatterning our breathing. This is because your body creates what's called nitric oxide when you breathe through your nose. Now, don't confuse this with the laughing gas they give you at the dentist's office—that's nitrous oxide.

Nitric oxide is produced naturally by your body and has a relaxing and calming effect, opening up your airways to promote more sustainable and unlabored breathing. It gives you access to your diaphragm, making it easier to breathe and leaving you with a calm disposition with the ability to respond to life instead of reacting.

Breathing during exercise becomes so much easier. You may discover you're moving better and that you have more energy during your workout, recovering much faster afterward.

You may even be able to do more without depleting yourself because you've improved your oxygen uptake by breathing predominately through your nose.

I've experienced this firsthand. I used to have exercise-induced asthma, and because of this, I've always hated high-intensity cardio. I still hate high-intensity cardio, but now I'm able to do it if I want to without compromising my breathing because I've trained myself to breathe through my nose. Therefore more efficiently taking in oxygen by retaining more carbon dioxide in my body.

Now, I'm not a doctor, but I really think that we could solve so many cases of sleep apnea and anxiety by just retraining people to breathe through their noses. Not to mention you'd forever know how much energy you have to devote to a workout or whatever you're wanting to do by just checking in with your breathing.

All due to just developing an ability to tap into our body's own natural technology—no drugs, just breathing. It is magical.

ACTION STEPS

Action Step 1

Try this simple breathing exercise: Have your stopwatch on hand. Start by taking a natural inhale. Hold it for a second and then exhale as slowly as you can and time how long it takes you to exhale all the air out.

If it's below fifteen seconds, this might be an indication your oxygen uptake is low at that moment, and you may want to gear your workout and activities according to that by paring them down a bit. If it's above fifteen seconds, then you're doing pretty good, and you have enough energy and oxygen uptake for a full workout.

This is a great tool to determine if you are still recovering from the day before and how much energy you have to afford for that day.

Action Step 2

Nose breathing awareness exercise: Begin by becoming aware of how much you breathe through your nose each day. Notice when you start breathing through your mouth. Is it when you're concentrating on something? When you're working at the computer? When you're walking or working out moderately? When you're watching TV?

Oftentimes, we become mouth-breathers when we are doing things without awareness. It's okay to mouth breathe during times when you are doing smaller intense bursts of exercise, but then I recommend you get back to nose breathing as soon as you can.

We become nose-breathers by closing our mouth, breathing through our nose, and then bringing the tongue to the rough of the mouth. This aids in reshaping the face and jaw area over time and then creates more space in the jaw.

I started this practice when I'd hike. I'd notice when in my hike I had to go to mouth breathing (usually going up a steep hill) and then switch over to nose breathing again as soon as I could. After a while, it became so much easier to maintain nose breathing through most of my hike, and then I was able to incorporate it into my day without even thinking about it.

Really all I'm doing is asking you to pay attention to how much you are nose breathing compared to mouth breathing each day, and then when you notice it, change it. That's all; that's your breathing practice. It's very simple. Just developing your awareness around this can take you so far.

CHAPTER 17

YOUR BODY
CRAVES LIGHT

YOUR PHYSICAL AND SUBTLE ENERGETIC BODY CRAVES LIGHT.
Much like plants, we need light to thrive. This can be explained
in a simple scientific concept called photosynthesis, a process
where all organisms convert light into energy.[2]

We all learn about photosynthesis in elementary school, yet
most of us don't know how to put this into practice when we
become adults. We need to expose ourselves to light from the
sun in healthy, small amounts every day. During the wintertime, if you live in a place where you don't get much sun, then
it's great to use light therapy in the form of red, yellow, and
orange spectrum light.

The light that we take in through our body aids in producing
key enzymes that will activate mitochondria in your cells and
produce energy. Mitochondria are the powerhouses of our cells.

---

2 "Photosynthesis," Wikipedia, last modified September 2, 2021, https://en.wikipedia.org/
wiki/Photosynthesis.

They aid in taking the energy we get from food and converting it into energy that the cell can access and use.[3]

It's truly incredible if you think about it. I can completely understand why, at one time, we worshiped the sun gods. The sun brings life to everything it touches. We need it to grow food; we need it to produce energy and thrive as human beings.

There's both a physical and an energetic component to this. You bring light to a situation. You can light someone up. You can draw light into your body to heal and energize it. You can enlighten someone with your insights and perspective. You can enlighten people by exposing your creativity. These are all things we say to each other casually, but do we really know that what we're saying is true in a sense?

We say these things because we feel them. When someone walks into a room and has the effect on you that feels as if you're instantly energized and inspired, that person has just lit you up. We do this for each other all the time. By bringing light into a situation, you open up possibilities and bring love into it.

Just as you can expose your physical body to light and have it respond by activating your mitochondria and producing energy, you can bring light into your body energetically when you meditate. This has a calming and grounding effect on your energy body, aiding you in clearing anything energetically that no longer serves you and filling in the space with pure love.

---

3 Tim Newman, "What Are Mitochondria?" *Medical News Today*, February 8, 2018, https:// www.medicalnewstoday.com/articles/320875.

ACTION STEPS

Action Step 1

Go back to the "connecting to the light" meditation, and do this daily or as needed.

Action Step 2

A quick way you can connect with the light is to imagine a white light waterfall coming down and filling the crown of your head with light and then filling up your entire body with a waterfall of loving light.

Action Step 3

Get a healthy daily dose of vitamin D by getting out in the sun. You can sunbathe for ten to fifteen minutes on each side of your body, or if you aren't exposed to sunlight in the wintertime, buy a red light and sit under it for ten to twenty minutes a day.

CHAPTER 18

A HEALTHY SPINE EQUALS A HEALTHY BODY

THE PHRASE "THE STRAW THAT BROKE THE CAMEL'S BACK" COMES from the proverb, "It's the last straw that breaks the camel's back." It describes this situation beautifully, meaning a minor or routine action that causes an unpredictably large and sudden reaction because of the cumulative effect of small actions.[4]

Back pain is one of those things that, if you've ever experienced it, you'll never forget it. If you've had a back spasm, there's a pretty good chance you're very fearful of having another one. It'll literally bring you to your knees.

I remember when I had my first back spasm. I'd never experienced anything like it before, so naturally, I had no idea what

---

4 "Straw that Broke the Camel's Back," Wikipedia, last modified June 23, 2021, https://en.wikipedia.org/wiki/Straw_that_broke_the_camel%27s_back.

was happening to me. All I did was bend over to try on a shoe at a local boutique and instantly felt my back tighten up like it never had before. It continued to progressively get worse as I started to quickly walk home. When I got home, I lay on the sofa for a while, then tried to get up to go to the bathroom, and a debilitating spasm stopped me in my tracks. I couldn't move. Panicked, I thought to myself, *what if I never walk again?* More immediately, how was I going to get to the bathroom?

It was terrifying. Looking back, it was also a time when I wasn't putting the missing pieces of my life together. This was one of the biggest lessons I learned from my back pain. I had to listen to what both my body and my soul were telling me. I wasn't listening. Instead, I was overriding my body's messages, one being what my heart was calling me to do.

And what was the message? No more people-pleasing and fitting in at the expense of myself. My back was telling me that we could no longer hold this anymore. The dam was about to break.

During this experience, I learned that our spine symbolizes safety, security, and stability in our life. Think about that. How emotionally secure and stable do you feel in your life? Do you feel safe in your body? Do you trust that the universe will take care of you?

I can say with confidence that, at that time, I didn't feel any of these things. The 2008 housing market crash had just hit, and my husband and I were heavily invested as Atlanta real estate developers. We were doing so well that we decided to up the ante and started to build new homes that would sell in the million-dollar price range. It could have gone either way. We could have walked away millionaires or lost everything. Unfortunately, it was the latter.

For the first time in my life, I felt like a financial failure. We filed for bankruptcy, we lost our house to foreclosure, and we watched as the cops prevented us from even taking our own fridge with us. It was a truly shameful experience. Luckily, we owned a very modest rental in the same neighborhood, and we were able to move into it. It was an old seventies duplex that we converted from a two-unit to a single-unit home by just taking out the wall between the two units.

We were able to make lemonade out of lemons.

In hindsight, it was a blessing because it allowed us to get rid of close to 90 percent of the stuff we had acquired over the years—stuff that didn't matter as much as we thought it did. We realized it definitely wasn't bringing us happiness, so why not try something different. A more minimalist approach, and so that's what we did.

The experience was liberating at first. We slowly let go of our dependence on "stuff" and went through a lengthy process of getting out of debt completely. This was our new mission in life: truly taking on the minimalist mindset.

Although I felt so free and I'd regained a sense of control when I started releasing all my material stuff, what I came to realize was that I needed to do some inner work before I could move on. My back pain was a clear reminder of this.

The good news is that, amidst all the chaos, we were able to figure out how to make it work. The only problem was that my whole inner world was changing, and I didn't even notice; I just kept going.

It was a spiritual crisis that was many years in the making. I'd lost all trust in the universe and how it could take care of me. I was left feeling like I had to do this all by myself, not realizing that I was *choosing* the hard way. There's nothing that will get your attention more than the feeling of not being supported in life.

I remember feeling like I had no control, much like I felt when my parents got divorced when I was a young teen. I felt like the rug was being pulled out from under me, leaving me with nothing to stand on when it was all said and done.

I was grasping for a sense of control, and when I couldn't find it, I tried controlling everything myself. No wonder my back went out. It was the last straw. You bend down to tie your shoe one day or you twist funny to pick up your kid, and your back goes out. You wonder where that came from, not realizing that it was a big reaction to many smaller actions over time.

In Louise Hay's book, *Heal Your Body*, she gives you the breakdown of all the segments of the spine and what it could mean on a deeper level to have pain and dysfunction in the spine and how it relates to your soul's messages. Louise also provides you affirmations and an idea of what could be going on emotionally and spiritually.

I love this because it brings in a deeper aspect and new dimension to our health. Not just the physical but also the energetic and how they interplay. Approaching your back from a practical standpoint, like assessing if you're sitting in one position too long, not moving enough, not eating well, or not sleeping enough, are all very important. There's also the question of if you're living a heartfelt, joyful life.

Like I mentioned earlier, your body is very intuitive. It knows how to get your attention.

My back pain represented old trauma, emotional pain, a sense of lack, victimhood, a false sense of control, and a lack of trust for some time. I was only able to get a handle on it when I began looking at it from all dimensions of reality. The physical, emotional, mental, and spiritual bodies, all parts of myself.

There's so much value in taking action within your physical form out of the need to get out of pain. If you truly wish to stay out of pain, you also have to approach the value in the energetic components of your life and how they interplay.

Once my clients are cleared by their doctors and therapists to work with me, I always teach them both how to identify what could be going on with their back if they ever get into pain again and teach them a movement routine they can use to get into balance with their back again.

These tools are essential. I also explain to them that if there is some kind of emotional, mental, or spiritual component, this can you slow down possibly in order to see a broader perspective.

This self-evaluation can be extremely valuable, and as we understand our body a little more, this begins to build trust back in ourselves without the fear of reinjury. Guidance is important, especially when you are the one that's in pain.

I learned how to do the right movement therapy and found an excellent chiropractor and physical therapist, both of whom I actually worked with too. I also hired my own personal trainer to hand over my observations of myself to someone who could give me a different perspective that I could learn from and trust without having to figure it all out by myself.

This got me out of pain and provided me with the physical stability and strength to do the work I needed to acknowledge my deeper emotional pain.

More importantly, I needed to address my relationship with money and the universe. It all relates to your ability to receive abundance in your life and how much you trust the universe to take care of you.

There is so much power in this kind of exploration. This, of course, is heavily influenced by how you received love and money from your parents. Although this is not a money book, it's important to bring it up because it seems to be a common factor in people with recurring back pain: safety and financial security.

Many people have a stressful relationship with love and money or a hard time receiving both. Back pain can also represent a spiritual conflict or going against what their spirit is calling them to do. In my case, it was a little bit of both. Like many people, I wasn't taught that there was a connection here until I experienced it firsthand. I also realize that there are so many aspects to back pain, and it's very dependent on the individual's personal experience. What I've learned is that if there's a discrepancy in these areas, you can get to the heart of the issue much faster by addressing the body's mental, emotional, and spiritual aspects.

Your energy will always manifest into your physical form, not vice versa, according to another powerful book, *Miracles Through Pranic Healing* by Master Choa Kok Sui. He states that manifestation begins in the subtle energy body with what he describes as thought entities and then manifests in the physical form as either disease or lasting health and wellness. This is why it all matters.

ACTION STEPS

Action Step 1

Mobility exercises—cat-cow articulation check-in and daily traction and open book upper back rotation: The best exercise I can think of to check in with your spine on a daily basis is called the cat-cow articulation. If you're familiar with the cat-cow move in yoga, you'll already be somewhat familiar with this one. The only difference is you are articulating each spinal segment instead of moving your back all at once.

Start on your hands and knees and begin by bringing your attention to your tailbone area. Begin by tucking it under and going up the spine one spinal segment at a time as slow as you can until you reach your head. Your head is the last to round down. Then you'll reverse this by again starting at the tailbone, lifting it up, going down each spinal segment until you reach the head, which will come up last. Repeat this at least five times.

Notice any stickiness, restrictions, tightness, or tenderness in any areas of the spine. How does it feel? Does this motion alone help your back move better? This will most likely help to both check in with your back and get more circulation and mobility to your spine. It's a win-win.

Go to www.finallythrivingbook.com to see these back exercises.

Action Step 2

Journal: Grab your pen and your journal and write five ways you like to be supported. Then begin practicing this by receiving that support in your life. For example, if someone wants to buy you a coffee or lunch, how would it feel to let them do that without you justifying it? How would it feel to receive the support and love you crave and be able to trust you are taken care of? Write that down too. It may feel messy and uncomfortable at first, and that's totally normal. Always remember this is a practice, so if you're out of practice with your receiving love and support, then there's the act of practicing how to receive in a way that serves everyone involved.

Once you begin to master the ability to receive, giving begins to feel natural because you learn how to give unconditionally. When your bucket is full, you have more than enough to go around, and you develop the desire to give to others because you know what it feels like to receive without conditions.

Scientific Support

Richard A. Brown, "Spinal Health: The Backbone of Chiropractic's Identity," *Journal of Chiropractic Humanities* 23, no. 1 (December 2016): 22–28, https://doi.org/10.1016/j.echu.2016.07.002.

CHAPTER 19

FREE YOUR FEET

OUR FEET CONNECT US TO THE GROUND WE ARE STANDING ON and are foundational to our health. Yet we rarely give them much consideration when it comes to our health and performance.

I've seen so many of my clients dumbfounded when they discover most of their hip and knee issues were due to their feet not moving properly under them.

Your feet are quite frankly what grounds you to the earth. This actually happens electromagnetically, and science can explain this. That's why just walking barefoot in the grass can lead to feeling better and more connected.

Unfortunately, even though they protect our feet and look fabulous, shoes can hinder our ability to get signals from the ground to your feet and other parts of your body. This can be an issue when you're walking over uneven terrain and your feet aren't given the opportunity to adapt and mold to it by moving properly over the ground. Your feet become these tight blocks under you that lack mobility.

Your feet have a unique sensory feedback because of this. Because it's so important to feel the ground we are stepping over. It's important from a practical standpoint so we can adapt to the ground we're stepping on with the rest of the body as well. The feet are taking all the impact and force many times. Treat your feet well.

If our feet aren't able to adapt, sensor, and mobilize over the ground we're stepping on, our knees have to take on the job of the feet, and they don't have the capacity to do it as well. So, as a result, we get knee, hip, and even back pain as a result of not properly freeing our feet.

According to Katy Bowman's book, *Move Your DNA*, your feet have lots of sensors that'll indicate what you're stepping over, allowing you to adjust the pressure with which you're stepping. We've lost the ability to connect with this sensory mechanism in our feet because of thick-soled, narrow-toed, and high-heeled shoes. Plus, we're mostly walking on flat concrete surfaces.

Otherwise, the signal that your feet are getting gets skewed and discombobulated, leading to a lack of awareness and feeling in our body. It's important to allow our feet to move over different terrains and feel the surface we're walking over to regain this sense of connection to both our body and the earth.

This can also lead to better balance. Since your feet are literally adapting to surfaces you walk or stand on, the better your feet are able to adapt, the better you'll be able to balance. The ability to balance is probably one of the most important skills to maintain as we get older.

Another way to check in with your feet is to look at how well your toes are moving. Can you spread your toes? Can you lift one toe up individually at a time?

Your toes are a really great indication of how well the muscles and bones are moving in your feet. You can quickly free your feet up by just implementing some regular toe stretching and foot mobilization as well as changing your shoe wear.

ACTION STEPS

Action Step 1

You can get started by walking barefoot in the grass and around your home. Buy shoes that have a thinner, more flexible sole and a wider toe box. Minimalist shoes will allow you to better feel the ground you're walking over.

Action Step 2

To mobilize your feet, take a lacrosse ball and lightly roll it under your foot. Do some ankle and toe stretching daily.

Go to www.finallythrivingbook.com for these foot exercises.

Action Step 3

Start a "walking practice." Walk thirty minutes or more daily.

Suggestions on how you can choose to experience your walk:

- Walk in nature. Observe and feel the energy around you.

- Make it a walking meditation with no distractions and no phone.

- Listen to music, a sound frequency, or guided meditation as you walk.

- Pay attention to your feet and gait as you are walking; swing your arms.

- Listen to an audiobook or podcast while you walk.

CHAPTER 20

HOW FLEXIBLE ARE YOU, BOTH LITERALLY AND FIGURATIVELY?

FEEL INTO YOUR BODY WHEN YOU STRETCH AND NOTICE THE tight spots. Notice where you hold tension in your body.

Is it in your spine? Is it in your hips? Is it in your neck? How mobile are your feet? Is there tension between your eyes?

Does it feel good to stretch this area? Is it painful or uncomfortable? Does it hold on for dear life, or can you feel it letting go? Are you enjoying the stretch? Does it feel good? Does it feel stable and supported?

These are all things to notice when you stretch. I have a sequence of dynamic and passive stretches I put all of my clients through in the beginning and end of every session we have together. I do this because I want them to consistently get to know their body this way.

I call it a daily body check-in where it gives them an opportunity to check in with their body and notice what needs attention, what feels good that day, or even what feels like it's improved.

This is so important because this teaches them how to listen to what their body is telling them. It'll tell them what direction to go in. We just have to learn how to pay attention.

By paying attention and giving your body that kind of time and priority, you send a message that it is important to you. Once you learn how to give your body the attention it needs, it'll respond beautifully and let you know what's going on. Plus, you'll have a much more enjoyable workout.

Flexibility can also be a reflection of how you're integrating your life. If you have many places of inflexibility in your body, ask yourself where you are resisting the goodness in life. What are you not wanting to pay attention to or change? What are you holding on to?

Pay attention to what you are tolerating in your life but that you really don't want to tolerate anymore. Be honest with yourself. Is it living on a busy street, the way people treat you, or the way you treat yourself?

Write these down, and see if there's anything you are willing to let go of to create more space to do more of what you really want to do, how you want to express yourself, and how you want to be living.

The other side of the coin is that tightness can mean there's a weakness in that area. Other times, activating your stabilizer muscles and learning how to strengthen your body will aid in creating more flexibility. If you're always stretching the same area and never making any progress, this could be what's going on.

And by all means, keep checking in and stretching your body. I love to stretch my body before I go to bed every night. If I'm watching a show, I'm on the floor stretching while I watch. It's really the best for winding down at the end of your day.

So what is the difference between passive stretching and dynamic stretching?

Passive stretching is when you hold a stretch for about sixty to ninety seconds. It's something I reserve for both the end of a workout and before I go to bed at night. Dynamic stretching, on the other hand, is a good thing to do at the beginning of your workout and throughout the day. It's more of a moving stretch getting to your end range comfortably but not pushing it as hard as you would in your passive stretch.

Dynamic stretching is best to use before your workout since it works to mobilize your body without shutting stability muscles off like passive stretching will do. This approach to stretching preps your body by safely exploring the end range of your movement and by activating your muscles for stability.

Passive stretching is great for training the body to go further by slowly lengthening the muscles while holding a stretch. This will sometimes create small tears in the muscles, similar to what happens when you lift weights. What results after repair is the muscle and connective tissue reshaping into a more lengthened position. This is how you create flexibility over time.

ACTION STEP

Try some dynamic and passive stretches.

Go to www.finallythrivingbook.com to access these stretches.

Scientific Support

"Benefits of Flexibility Exercises," *Harvard Health Publishing*, April 16, 2015, https://www.health.harvard.edu/staying-healthy/benefits-of-flexibility-exercises.

CHAPTER 21

GET TO KNOW YOUR PERSONAL RHYTHM

WHAT IS YOUR PERSONAL RHYTHM?

When does it suit you to work out?

What time of day do you prefer to eat?

Do you set it, or do outside sources dictate your rhythm?

Your personal rhythm is how you set the tone for your day. It is, essentially, your daily routine. Do you go back and forth feeling like your day is scattered, or is there an organized structure and flow to your day?

Our personal rhythm is incredibly important when it comes to how we cultivate and utilize our energy. A structured daily routine will nurture and expand our energy; a nonexistent or erratic routine is going to diminish our energy. Depending on your day-to-day experience, you can probably feel in your body which one is accurate for you.

Your body has something called an organ body clock. This concept is rooted in traditional Chinese Medicine and is based on the time of day your chi or life force energy flows through each organ and energizes it. You can intuitively feel into this, although it's just as helpful to look at a map of your organ body clock. You can find this in the book *The Body Clock in Traditional Chinese Medicine* by Lothar Ursinus.

Are you running around from task to task, staying busy all day, and leaving nothing for yourself at the end of the day? Is your energy spent, with nothing to show for it but exhaustion? When we live life this way, we find ourselves always wondering where the time goes and maybe even beating ourselves up for not treating our hearts and bodies better.

Honoring your personal rhythm is an act of self-discipline that gives you back to yourself. It's a way for you to reclaim your personal time and also be of service to others in a way that nourishes you. If you want to avoid energy depletion and stay clear and grounded in your own purpose and intention, you must discover your personal rhythm and dedicate yourself to it.

Where do we begin? It all starts with your meals. Your meals dictate your energy flow for the day, and I don't just mean what you're eating. Making sure you're setting aside ample time for preparing your food and eating peacefully is equally important. Eating meals should be considered "downtime," not a time to get an extra task done.

Make time for yourself first thing in the morning. Start with breakfast and then get your meditation or walk in before you start your day. Prepare your intention for what you'll do that day. Look at your to-do list. Is it way too much or very doable? Ask your soul what it would like to do today, and then honor that. There's no wrong answer.

It's also about the time of day you devote to your daily movement. There are so many different schools of thought out there about this, but in my opinion, getting to know your personal rhythm will dictate the most optimal time to honor your movement practice.

I've discovered my own personal rhythm is stretching and walking in the morning after I've had my breakfast and a good bowel movement. I'll then reserve my workout for later in the morning or midday. I find that I have more energy to access at that time, and my body feels better when I work out fully awake.

It's also good to consider if you're in a low energy state, how your thyroid is responding to your life, and how you're recovering and sleeping. If you're having any issues related to what I just mentioned, I've found it better for most people to work out or do light exercise mid-morning or midday.

As the day goes on, it's more important to wind your body down instead of amping it up. This rhythm will eventually affect your sleep cycle.

When I'm able to get a nice walk in after breakfast and then a short meditation, it leaves me feeling more aligned, so I'm able to step into my own energy before I start my day. That way, I have the time and space to spend with my clients and time in the middle of the day for my own needs. I'm then able to wind down in the evening feeling fully relaxed.

I have a routine that doesn't stress me out or leave me feeling like I've done too much without replenishing myself.

When we don't give time to ourselves, we can end the day feeling irritated, annoyed, frustrated, and unable to prioritize ourselves. It leaves you tense and quite frankly anxious. After a while, you build up resentment toward others, and you're left wondering where this is all coming from. It's coming from a place of not honoring your personal rhythm.

Everyone is different. Some people can do many things at once and still have time for themselves without any stress. Others need only a few tasks a day; otherwise, they feel overwhelmed and can't reserve time for themselves.

Which category do you fall under? Over the years, I've found that I really need a few consistent things to do each day; otherwise, I'll overdo it and then my energy tanks.

Over-scheduling myself will initially look doable on a calendar but then actually following through becomes very time-consuming. More times than not, I'll underestimate the energy I'll have to put into a meeting.

So that's why my motto now is doing less is more. Plus, I only do things for work that are enjoyable to me. Doing things that are enjoyable will generate more energy for me in the short and long term.

When you expend energy on doing what you love, this naturally energizes you. So doing what you're passionate about affords you the ability to do more without excess energy expenditure. This is possible and very doable. I think that's because as we begin to bring more awareness to where we siphon our energy, we're able to put our energy toward things that will energize us more instead of depleting us.

My advice is to make certain you do things you enjoy and desire to work toward a practice. It'll benefit you more because then you'll be able to see how it consistently pays off, and you're better able to get to know your own daily rhythm.

ACTION STEPS

Action Step 1

Tune in each morning and ask your soul what it would like to do that day. Write your answer down, and then at the end of each day, see if you honored that. How did it feel when you honored that? How did it feel when you didn't honor that?

Action Step 2

Look at your schedule and notice how you feel when you look at it. Does it feel joyful, light, and fun, or does it feel heavy, obligated, and stifling?

Action Step 3

Take off anything that you no longer want to obligate yourself to. Notice if your schedule makes sense for you and matches your natural rhythm.

CHAPTER 22

LIVE DIRTY
AND EAT CLEAN

THERE'S A LEVEL OF DIRTINESS THAT WE MUST MAINTAIN TO stay healthy and balanced.

Our bodies are a reflection of what we see in nature, so just like the soil, we must have a nice variable terrain of bacteria both in and on our body—more specifically, in your gut and on your skin. This is your superpower, and it's a part of what makes you human.

The notion of over-sanitizing everything you come across has been severely misunderstood. We've been misinformed when it comes to cleanliness.

It's spectacular when you think about how our gut is a mirror of the dirt we grow our food in. Yet many of us don't realize that killing off all of the bacteria and fungi will kill the life force right out of the soil. The same goes for your body.

The simple truth is that soil from the Earth works a lot like what we call your gut microbiome. It needs a certain level of permaculture to thrive. All the fungus, bacteria, and weeds work together to grow some amazing food. The Earth makes compost, much like your body makes compost when you eliminate waste.

The notion of living dirty and eating clean makes so much more sense to me. When we're young, we must literally play in the dirt to build up a certain level of immunity and resilience in our bodies. This sets the stage for your health in your adult life.

If you've ever had a baby or been around babies, you'll notice that they put everything in their mouths, and in many other countries, babies and toddlers are left to play in the dirt and even eat it from time to time. The belief is that this will aid in building up a child's innate immune system and provide the gut with a plethora of good bacteria for the gut microbiome.[5]

Unfortunately, this wisdom has been lost, and we're now inundated with pharmaceuticals, GMOs, pesticides, chemical sanitizers, and the list goes on. Of course, we do have a certain level of resilience for our environment, but we get into trouble when there's an overload of toxicity that the body can no longer sift through. This is why it's important to know how to lighten your toxic load.

---

5 Noreen Iftikhar, "Baby Mouthing—AKA Why Do Babies Put Everything in Their Mouths?" *Healthline*, October 16, 2020, https://www.healthline.com/health/baby/baby-mouthing#reasons.

This is where living dirty and eating clean come into play. You can most easily lighten your toxic load first by eating clean. I'm sure you've heard that before, but many of us may wonder what that means.

What this means to me is that you're supporting the local farmers who are growing organic or pesticide-free foods and are feeding their animals what animals are meant to eat, like grass, bugs, and mushrooms.

These farmers practice regenerative farming, which helps the land regenerate instead of depleting the soil with chemicals and GMO grains. Eugene Trufkin's book, *Anti-Factory Farm Shopping Guide*, is a great resource for knowing what to look for when you shop. He goes into great detail about what the labeling means and how to find the cleanest, most optimal foods.

If you're interested in learning more about the practice of regenerative farming, Robb Wolf's book, *Sacred Cow*, explains how regenerative farming is better for the environment and your body. I also recommend reading Joel Salatin's book, *Folks, This Ain't Normal*. Joel is a farmer, speaker, and writer who has worked for decades to bring the art of permaculture farming back to the people by showing and teaching them how it's done.

In his book, he explains what permaculture is and how it's what nature intended, affording more healthy, clean food than we could ever imagine. He points out that we're doing it wrong with factory farming methods and that by bringing permaculture farming practices back, we can heal the Earth and have an unlimited food source without all the harmful chemicals. He shares that nature thrives symbiotically in a permaculture environment.

Joel's point is that what we are currently doing is not normal, and instead of working with nature, we're working against her and, in the process, making people sick.

This leads us right back to the soil. If our soil is not healthy, we'll not be able to grow nutrient-dense food, and the Earth will continue to degrade instead of naturally regenerating like it's supposed to.

Our bodies are not hard drives or machines; they are a part of nature. Yet if we fail to see ourselves this way, we lose the ability to connect to nature and reflect within ourselves what we see outside of ourselves. Our bodies are an incredibly intelligent force, and if you pay attention to what nature provides, you'll begin to see the many wonders your body provides too.

ACTION STEPS

Action Step 1

My advice is to start by supporting your local farmers. The people who are practicing regenerative farming, organic farming, or chemical-free farming. You just have to seek out and ask.

Show up at your local farmers' market and talk to the farmers about how they farm. Organic certification is best, but it's too expensive to get organic certification for some farmers, so some will farm under those principles or farm chemical-free without the certification. That's why asking is so important.

Action Step 2

Another way you can learn about this is to get Eugene's book, *Anti-Factory Farm Shopping Guide,* where he goes into great detail on how to find these optimal foods in your local grocery store. Take it with you to the grocery store and use it to decode the labeling they place on products so that you can find the most optimal foods for your body.

Action Step 3

If you want to take it one step further, create a more intimate relationship with your food by growing it in your backyard. If you are new to this, start your backyard garden with something that is easy to grow, like tomatoes, and watch them grow every day. You can even plant a fruit tree, which is my personal favorite. Take a moment to observe how different it is to pick food from your backyard garden. How does this feel compared to picking your food up at the grocery store?

Scientific Support

Katia Moskvitch, "Can You Be Too Clean?" *BBC*, November 19, 2015, https://www.bbc.com/future/article/20151118-can-you-be-too-clean.

CHAPTER 23

HORMONAL BALANCE

IF YOU WERE TO ASK ME WHAT THE TWO MOST OVERLOOKED aspects of health are, I'd without a doubt say blood sugar regulation and hormonal balance. I'm really not sure why hormones don't get enough consideration as something that could be out of balance. Maybe it's because they're misunderstood.

My perspective tends to lean more toward the easier route when it comes to hormonal balance.

If you don't make it too complicated by overanalyzing it or let your doctor take full control by giving you estrogen when you've reached menopause, then you're halfway there.

It's really very simple in my experience, but we make it super complicated. Now, full disclosure, I'm not an endocrinologist, so please take my advice with a grain of salt, and please, by all means, come to your own conclusions.

What I've learned is about gut health, proper blood sugar regulation, and liver function. If you take care of these, you're well on your way to healthy balanced hormones.

One reason I think hormones have become hard to understand is that we've misunderstood the roles of estrogen and progesterone in our body's processes.

Estrogen is not a female-only hormone because men and others have some levels of it too. However, estrogen plays a larger role for women and others who were assigned female at birth, as it kills off cells through a surge that causes a shedding effect in the uterus every month during menstruation. Estrogen creates an excitatory effect in the cells, and this causes the cells to die.

It's normal as a woman or person with a uterus to have an estrogen surge once a month when you're still menstruating. What's not normal is to have excess estrogen surges all of the time.

During menstruation, an initial estrogen surge excites the cells, killing off and shedding the cells; progesterone comes in after and helps to detox the excess estrogen from the gut and out the intestines. This is our natural process when we're in balance.

Because we live in constant stress mode, eat foods high in soy and polyunsaturated fats, suppress our trauma and emotions, move very little during the day, have poor blood sugar regulation, take in lots of toxins through our products like makeup and lotions, and don't rest or sleep enough, we find ourselves in a state of imbalance and estrogen dominance.

Instead of getting excreted through the intestines, the estrogen begins to recirculate through the intestines and into the body. It comes back to your liver, giving it more to work through.

Your liver is what converts your thyroid hormone, so if it's not happy, nobody's happy.

ACTION STEPS

Action Step 1

What can you do to avoid this? Start eating smaller, more frequent meals. Notice if you are going through a stressful state. A stressful state can be emotional, physical, environmental, or spiritual. Your body treats all stress the same, so the name of the game is to keep your metabolism running strong.

We do this by not letting our digestion get too slow and sluggish. If you're experiencing this, eat foods that are easy to digest, like bone broth, cooked veggies, cooked fruits, and slow-cooked meats. This process will break down your food so that you don't have to break it down while you're healing and getting your metabolism back on track.

Progesterone plays a very important role, too, as it favors pregnancy and is also a youth steroid hormone, which has an anti-inflammatory effect.

You can gain an ability to produce more progesterone by including certain foods in your diet: fruit like nectarines, papaya, tropical fruits, foods rich in fat-soluble vitamins like A and D, and sunlight.

Contrary to popular thought, good sugars can be therapeutic for your liver. Your liver literally runs on glucose. It depends on it and needs glucose to convert thyroid hormone. Your thyroid is the master regulator of your metabolism, so you can see how important it is for energy and ATP production in your mitochondria.

When your liver runs low on glucose, it'll get sluggish, and then your body will begin producing stress hormones to get you back up to that desired energy state. This only works for a short time. Over time, if you become dependent on stress hormones for energy, you lose your ability to produce energy efficiently with food, which aids the mitochondria in producing ATP.

I've said it before, and I'll say it again. The best thing you can do for yourself if you find yourself in this situation is to learn how to balance your blood sugar with a combination of the right amount of carbohydrates, proteins, and saturated fats. Although recommended serving sizes are usually different for everyone, you can start with one serving of each.

Action Step 2

Use a raw carrot to detox excess estrogen from your intestines. I first learned about this technique from Dr. Ray Peat. He explains how the carrot's antifungal properties and naturally absorbing fibers have the ability to pull out excess estrogen and endotoxins in the gut. This makes it a perfect tool for sterilizing the gut and detoxing. He even has a recipe for a carrot salad you can eat daily, which is both simple to make and delicious.

I love this because, like I've said before, it's not complicated unless we make it that way. Your body knows what to do; you just have to give it what it needs.

CHAPTER 24

WHY FOOD QUALITY MATTERS

I REMEMBER BACK WHEN I FIRST STARTED TEACHING MY CLIENTS that organic food was different from conventional food, and they'd look at me like I'd just told them that the Earth was flat.

In all honesty, even though it's pretty well known now that organic is better, I still find that there's this stigma about paying more for your food. I even get asked from time to time if GMOs are really a thing and if it's worth the extra money to avoid these.

Even more surprising is that the price between organic and non-organic food ends up evening out since many factory farms are subsidized. This means the taxpayer takes the brunt of the cost of the so-called cheaper nonorganic foods. This is the rub.

Now, for the most part, "organic" is a completely accepted idea thanks to Whole Foods Market, but it took years of teaching people the difference in their foods and marketing to change minds, even though some of the population has been psychologically tricked into thinking that organic foods are only reserved for the privileged people. Many continue to realize the value of the experience in going to your local farmers' market and the health benefits from eating high-quality foods.

Again, if we realize how these GMOs and junk foods are being subsidized and even compare prices, we soon realize we're actually getting a better deal by buying high-quality, organic foods. It's a win-win because you're supporting your local farmers, the regeneration of the Earth, and your body. Better yet, one of the best side effects of eating higher-quality foods is you need less medical intervention, and you feel great. Ultimately, you end up paying less in medical bills, which goes a long way these days.

Buying organic is cheaper.

Marketing to people in favor of high-quality foods is something I'm all for. Whole Foods, in its early years, was a pioneer in supporting local farms and highlighting them, whereas we had essentially lost our connection with where our food was coming from before this.

Gone were the days when your local dairy would drop off your fresh unpasteurized milk at your doorstep. With the rise of industrial farming and GMOs, the connection between the farmer and the consumer almost went away completely.

Thank goodness for people like Joel Salatin bringing permaculture back and other farmers who support regenerative farming. These people teach us the difference between food grown in a monocrop and food that's grown in a more diverse permaculture, or animals brought up in feedlots as opposed to animals brought up in a diverse environment free to roam. The latter being what nature intended.

Joel Salatin literally demonstrates this at his farm in Virginia. His mission was to show people how nature works synergistically. For example, the cows eat the grass, then they poop on the grass, and the worms and bugs eat the poop, and the chickens come behind and eat the worms and the bugs. The poop also naturally fertilizes the plants. This is a very simplified view of how permaculture works, but you get the point. Mother Nature knows what she's doing.

When we try to intervene with Mother Nature to the extent we have, we're changing our health, how we respond to our natural environment, and our relationship with nature.

This is big. I almost cannot fathom the level at which this is taking us away from our natural state of health and well-being. It all starts with your relationship with food and trickles down into your relationship with nature.

The truth is, you are nature, and whether you believe it or not, you are affected by it. So why not start healing your relationship with nature today? Because ultimately, you are healing your relationship with yourself.

Start by getting to know the farms that are local to where you live. In Eugene Trufkin's book, *Anti-Factory Farm Shopping Guide*, he teaches you how to identify a regenerative farming approach and differentiate between those products and a factory farming product in your local supermarket.

This is a great place to start. Educate yourself on the language that food companies use to market foods to you. I love Eugene's book because he makes something as complicated as the food industry's marketing lingo simple and easy to understand for the layperson.

I believe it's made complicated and less straightforward for a reason. Most companies want to take the less expensive route if they can get away with it, using low-grade ingredients like canola oil and soy to lengthen shelf life and then slapping a label on it like "All Natural."

It's about as far from "All Natural" as it gets, but since that sounds really good to the consumer, they'll buy it without question. Just remember, the food industry is not looking out for your best interests; they ultimately want to make a profit. They'd only listen and change their ways if people didn't buy their products and instead demanded something better—believe me.

Some companies are doing it right, and those are the ones I like to support. Educating yourself on what food quality is and the companies that actually care about it is paramount.

ACTION STEPS

Action Step 1

Make a list of farms that are local to you. Go talk to them.

Action Step 2

Educate yourself on the language that food companies use to market to you.

Action Step 3

Always read your food labels—become aware of what you are buying and who you are supporting.

CHAPTER 25

GET YOUR NUTRITION ON TRACK

Is your nutrition on track? Are you able to feel when your nutrition is off track?

It seems obvious that we'd know when our nutrition is off track, but it's actually not that obvious to many of us because we've never really been taught how to decode what our body is telling us.

How you respond to your life is a big clue. A healthy, optimistic disposition can be the first sign that your nutrition is on track.

This one is not as easy to identify. I've really had to ponder over the years and dig deep into what that really means and how to use discernment around it.

There's a difference between denying how you truly feel by stuffing your feelings and feeling healthily optimistic. Having optimism just means you're open to new possibilities. It's like starting the day from the point of view of a curious child excited about what they'll discover. It's a feeling of natural joy and curiosity about the world. You have abundant, joyful energy.

The other side of this is waking up every day dreading your life, always circling back to a state of learned helplessness, or overriding your feelings because of fear of being seen, feeling vulnerable, feeling pain, etc. You may even go so far as to act like everything's okay, denying your shadow parts.

Let's get into the psychology of it, but first, let's acknowledge that our psychology also depends on our body's physiology. This is how I want to share with you that nutrition can play an easy part in a healthy psychology.

If we're managing our blood sugar by eating regular meals and not leaving out any macronutrients (carbohydrates, protein, and fat), we're setting our body up for success, like getting a full night of sleep. This is optimal health. Allowing our body to do its job by supporting and learning how to listen to it.

Addressing the season is important, as wintertime tends to be hardest on our physiology and, for many people, leads to seasonal depression or sickness. Looking at nutrient deficiency is an easy fix for someone who's suffering from this.

Becoming aware of our body's signals that our nutrition is off track in the first place is crucial; otherwise, we go down the road of antidepressant medication, and the list goes on.

Let's look at the signs that your nutrition is off track. These aren't exactly obvious to most people, but there are some that I've put together over the years from working with countless clients and signs I've noticed within myself—some of which I've identified as being the most important and easiest to address.

ACTION STEPS

Action Step 1

Get your nutrition on track checklist:

#1. A Healthy Disposition

As I mentioned earlier, a healthy disposition when you wake up in the morning is important to pay attention to. Again, this doesn't mean you fake it till you make it. It means you have a feeling of natural optimism. This is an indication you have good energy production and your thyroid is working properly. You're motivated and curious about discovering what the day may bring.

#2. Abundant Energy

Now, this one can get confused with overproducing adrenaline and cortisol. If you're running on stress hormones all of the time, you won't be running on energy that's sustainable. If you have abundant energy production with food, you have enough energy to do what you want in life. You're able to take care of yourself and live your dream, and you have the energy to give to others. This includes service and giving to others, contributing to your community, parenting, etc.

Your sexual drive is a good indicator of your energy levels too. You want to pay attention to your level of motivation and arousal because the first thing to go when our energy tanks is our sex drive. You aren't going to be relaxed enough to be intimate with someone if you've been in survivor mode and then find yourself exhausted.

Personally, I noticed I had low energy and was running on stress hormones when I lost my motivation to have sex. I was having a hard time getting aroused, and that wasn't something I'd ever experienced before. This first happened after I gave birth to my two sons, which was totally normal, but then later it hit me again after I'd recovered from my back injury and had gone through some stressful times emotionally. It was obvious to me that my low libido was due to my recovery, but I didn't realize that it was also a sign that I was severely energetically and hormonally depleted.

My body was telling me that it couldn't muster enough energy to relax enough to enjoy some good sex, so it wasn't going to work until I fully recovered and replenished with the right nutrients. I needed to build my energy back up so I could enjoy my life.

What I realized in that moment was that it was not obvious to me how simple the fix could be. My guess is that so many other women could be feeling this too. Because when you're in it, it's hard to pinpoint what could be happening and what needs to change.

Another sign of low energy could be that you get irritated very easily and feel like everyone is encroaching on your space. This is a good indication you aren't giving yourself enough time and energy. You have a short fuse and can only react to a situation in the moment enough to sidestep it, rather than in a conscious way, because you just don't have the energy to deal with it.

#3. Regenerative Capacity

Your ability to recover well is a big one. When you have enough energy, your ability to recover and regenerate is swift. Your injuries may not heal as fast as Wolverine's do, but they do heal at a natural rate.

You're recovering from your workouts without much soreness or none at all. You don't get sick too often, and you're not sick for very long when you do. You're not seeing signs of premature aging like muscle deterioration, hair loss, excessive wrinkles, acne, low libido, etc., and you're sleeping soundly throughout the night.

Your ability to regenerate your cells is a reflection of the level of energy your body has to devote to that. For example, your body will always put your organs first before it clears up acne because keeping your liver working is way more important than clear skin. It's about survival at that point, and we don't want to just survive; we want to thrive. To thrive, you must have more energy to work with.

Something I always pay attention to very closely is how my clients recover from their workouts. For many of us, our first introduction to fitness was the myth of "no pain, no gain," and although there's a small grain of truth to that statement, we often take it too far.

You can definitely have a ton of gain from no pain. Since most people experience pain as beginners in exercise, I prefer to go slow with the intensity factor and gradually move them up to levels they can handle. Thus giving my first-time exercisers the foundation to lay the harder work later. As you become more experienced in exercise, you'll find you won't get sore as often.

When you justify excessive soreness in the name of getting "in shape," it's an indication that you do not have the energy to recover at the rate you're working out. You must slow your roll.

I always teach my clients how to pay attention to this as so many of them have been taught that pain after a workout means you had a good workout.

What this actually means is that you have a buildup of lactic acid in your body. This often leads to chronic inflammation if it's not acknowledged. It's very much like getting a sunburn. You won't ruin your skin if you get one or two sunburns in your lifetime, but if you continue to do it every summer, you'll end up with aging skin that is not healthy.

You've overly stressed your system and created a constant inflammatory response that your body now has to devote precious energy and resources to recover from.

It's okay and totally normal to have moderate muscular pain after you've done something for the first or second time, but there's a difference between that and not being able to sit on the toilet the next day. The soreness should subside for the most part as you train and get stronger. Soreness to that extreme just means you went too far and that you are not giving your body enough time to recover between workouts.

We're breaking the muscle down when we lift weights, and then there's the potential for the muscle to repair and build up. That's how it works, so you want to do this gradually in a way that your body can handle and adapt to over time.

If you are new to exercise, you may get sore in the beginning, and that's totally normal. Give yourself time to recover and use your recovery tools like your foam rolling and stretching. Epsom salt baths work wonders for recovering sore muscles.

As you get stronger, learn how to mobilize and recover; you'll soon find that you won't get sore as often or at all anymore.

In order to understand how we support our body in this process, we have to understand how our bodies work at the cellular level. Simply put, energy maintains structure and function at your body's cellular level.

Since your body depends on a constant energy source for structure and function, not fueling your body with enough frequency and with accessible nutrients will lead to structural degeneration in your body. Meaning connective tissue inflammation and breakdown.

If we look at how your body regulates your temperature, circulation, mood, and ability to recover from stress, we can figure out

149

what your body is missing. Once you discover this, it can only lead to a faster recovery, more energy, a positive outlook on life, and more joy.

We run into problems if we continue to use more energy than we take in. Issues like fatigue, autoimmune response, inflammation, nagging injuries, a slow metabolism, slow digestive motility, depression, weight gain, and more. It doesn't matter if the energy is used in a workout or sitting at the computer; it's all the same to your body because you're using energy for all of it. Even as I write this book, I'm using more brain energy to do it as opposed to if I were training my body. Sitting at the computer also strains your eyes and taxes your brain in a way that makes it harder to recognize when you are getting fatigued.

When it comes to aging, your body has bigger priorities than hair loss, gray hair, or wrinkles. Your body will conserve your energy and use it for more important jobs like pumping the heart and feeding the brain.

A body that's low in energy and not receiving the nourishment to recover will stay in a constant state of inflammation or injury. But if you have the energy reserves to make new tissue, your aging slows, and your injuries and inflammation get better because your body now has something to work with.

I remember a time when I was in the so-called "best shape" of my life and felt miserable. It was when I trained for a bodybuilding competition. I was in my early twenties, retired from gymnastics, and wanting something physically and mentally challenging. I'll admit I probably didn't go about it the best way. At that time, I didn't know what I know now about nutrition, and I found myself using nutrition recommendations from bodybuilding magazines. I ended up depleted energetically and nutritionally with nothing left to give.

As a young mom in my early thirties, I decided to go on the antifungal diet because of some painful digestive distress I'd been under. This diet was extreme and very restrictive. At first, I felt great, but then I started to feel tired and depressed. My energy levels dropped big time, and I felt as though I'd hit severe chronic fatigue. I had to take naps every day and didn't feel like I could even play with my kids.

Finally, when I was at my wit's end, I got turned onto a new way of looking at nutrition after I began studying and started to really understand how the body worked at the cellular level. I found that life can be so much easier if you support your body in its natural processes, allowing your body to do its job better. I did intensive research and tested ideas on myself, and when they worked, I shared my practices with my clients.

As a result, I've seen phenomenal results from both myself and countless others. I soon felt I had a new zest for life, more energy, and the capacity to do more without depleting myself. Just by making it simple.

Getting to know your own body's physiology and nutrient needs will give you a clear direction and create focused, specific steps you can take to create a body you feel great in.

So how do we support this practically and integrate it into our lives?

We integrate this with a daily movement practice, a rest and recovery plan, proper blood sugar regulation, high-quality food, and repatterned breathing.

We also learn how to measure our physiological feedback.

One of the most accessible tools I use to gauge my physiological feedback is to check in with my temperature and pulse. If we use these tools to measure our physiological feedback, we can begin to understand what our patterns could be and how to improve our metabolism.

Measuring basal body temperature and pulse gives you information and feedback about the efficiency and strength of your metabolic function. These measurements can give you direct feedback on how well your body is able to heat itself and transport oxygen and nutrients to the cells in your body.

Broda Barnes, MD, who wrote, *Hypothyroidism, an Unsuspected Illness*, measured body temperature to determine subclinical hypothyroidism, which does not show up in standard blood chemistry tests. The thyroid regulates the metabolic furnace of the body—creating heat or controlling temperature. Your thyroid is the master regulator of your metabolism.

The basal body temperature originated from Dr. Broda Barnes when he discovered that hypothyroidism was being severely underdiagnosed in the medical community. He later developed a diagnostic test that was intended for thyroid function, and it became known as the "Barnes Basal Temperature Test."

This low-tech way of testing the strength of your metabolism can be a valuable, effective, and accessible tool. Measure your pulse by taking two fingers to your carotid artery on your neck and feeling for a strong pulse. Hold there for ten seconds, counting the beats, and then multiply that number by six (or hold it for a full sixty seconds) to get your full heartbeats per minute (bpm) measurement.

I recommend taking your temperature with an oral thermometer. Your optimum temperature will range between 97.8–98.6 °F or 36.6–37.0 °C. A normal rhythm should be reflected by a lower measurement in the morning and rise to its peak in midday and then decline in the evening. Your optimum pulse will range between 75–85 bpm at rest.

This will give you a good idea of how well your thyroid is heating your body up and if it's circulating enough to get crucial nutrients and oxygen to the tissues.

Action Step 2

Measure your physiological feedback: Start by taking your temperature and pulse first thing when you wake up in the morning, then thirty to forty-five minutes after breakfast, and then thirty to forty-five minutes after lunch. Taking your temperature and pulse first thing in the morning before you get out of bed will give you your true resting temperature and pulse. Taking it thirty to forty-five minutes after breakfast and lunch will give your metabolism sufficient time to regulate after you eat. You can take it consecutively for a week; this will give you a good indication of how well your metabolism is functioning.

Considerations for accurate readings:

- Women should avoid taking their temperature during ovulation when the temperature rises. Make sure you take both temperature and pulse measurements; don't leave out one or the other. Both measurements are measured to determine your thyroid function more accurately. This is the best way to see your metabolic pattern and determine if you are efficiently producing energy.

- Do not do this test when you are sick since any kind of stress, including illness, can lower thyroid function. Also, a fever could raise your normally low temperature and give you a faulty reading.

- If you're taking prescription drugs (especially antide-pressants), be aware that some drugs can affect your temperature and pulse. Because of this, I suggest taking your temperature and pulse at a different time than when you take your medication.

CHAPTER 26

USE YOUR INTUITION WITH YOUR NUTRITION

YOUR INTUITION WILL ALWAYS LEAD YOU TO WHAT YOUR BODY needs. This is the basis for the intuitive eating movement—an idea introduced by nutritionists Evelyn Tribole and Elyse Resch back in 1995—that encourages us to let go of strict guidelines and eat what and how our body wants. By honoring natural hunger cues and making peace with our food, our nutrition becomes second nature. The big question is: are you in alignment with your intuition? Learning how to decode the signals your body is uniquely sending you will help you better connect to your intuitive body.

For example, when my skin gets super dry and broken out, even if I rest and do all the things I need to do to recover properly, I know I might have a vitamin A deficiency. The best way to tell if you're lacking in something essential is to eat something rich in that mineral. So if I eat foods high in vitamin A—like oysters or liver—and I feel instantly better and see an improvement in my skin, I know that's probably what the issue was. This is how intuitive eating works.

Typically, though, when we think we're lacking in certain vitamins and minerals, we reach for supplements instead of whole foods. This is normal, considering we've all been conditioned to look for the "magic pill" to heal and sustain. The good news is there is a magic answer, but it's not a supplement; it's whole foods.

Nature didn't send us supplements. She gave us foods rich in precious vitamins and minerals that come in a complete and perfect package giving our bodies everything they need to thrive. Supplements are engineered, and, no matter how ethically made, they can leave you severely depleted of other nutrients since our body needs other vitamins and minerals to be taken in with that supplement to aid in absorption and assimilation. This is why it doesn't always work. Most people are not laying a good food foundation before implementing the supplementation and instead are expecting supplements to create a framework and foundation that only food can provide.

This is why I stress food first and why I encourage intuitive eating over any other self-prescribed diet. If you *need* to supplement after you've done the work of creating a solid food foundation, then you'll know it. But if you supplement before you build your food foundation, you'll never know what truly works for you and what doesn't, and you'll be hindering your ability to "hear" your body.

How do we become more intuitive with our food?

It begins by learning how to balance our blood sugar. This becomes a practice of getting to know your food patterns, your food timing and intake, and how that relates to your energy. Once you learn this valuable skill, you can begin to optimize your eating for more energy production. It will feel very technical at first but will get easier and easier. The goal is to set a strong foundation so that nutrition becomes a pleasure and joy instead of a painful process of guessing and failing.

As you implement balancing your blood sugar, the next step is to move toward nutritious and delicious foods. The perceived deliciousness of food is important because if you're not enjoying your food, you won't produce the precious enzymes and saliva essential for your digestion.

This often gets skipped over in an attempt to sell people a program that is purely the most optimal food for health, but if the food is not delicious and delightful to the person, there's not much health benefit. This also goes for if the protocol is too strict. There won't be that much "buy-in" because there's no joy in the process.

This could be why so many nutrition programs only work for a short time and then stop working. It's not joyful, fun, or pleasurable to the person doing it. If you're not having fun in your program, then what's the point? I believe that getting healthy is learning how to create relaxation and joy in the body.

If you're creating more stress and restriction, then I'd ask if this is the right program for you.

It goes without saying that you are also learning new skills and putting these into practice. There's a period within this to have enough discipline to learn what's right for you and follow through with inspired action.

What's been misconstrued is that healthy eating has to be difficult, and if it's too pleasurable, you're doing something wrong or being overindulgent.

Eating delicious foods doesn't mean you're a bad person. It just means you're enjoying your food. This leads to more relaxation in the body and better digestion overall. It means that you are hitting the mark and tapping into your best self. Learning how to digest life in a beautiful way.

If you're not finding joy in your process, you may want to rethink it. I invite you to discover the intersection between delicious and nutritious.

ACTION STEPS

Eat by candlelight to create a more relaxing mood when you eat.

Make sure your food is both nutritious and delicious.

Eat without distractions, like TV or computer time.

CHAPTER 27

YOUR MAGICAL
IMMUNE SYSTEM

"We are not defined 'somas' produced once by our DNA, but rather adaptive, epigenetic, ongoing creative beings."

—Dr. Ray Peat

YOUR IMMUNE SYSTEM IS NOT A ONE-TRICK PONY. IT HAS THE ability to be extremely adaptive and creative in how it responds to the world. Yet we've just forgotten this. We've forgotten just how creative our body can be, mainly because we're always trying to control it and intervene.

In Dr. Ray Peat's article, "This Novel Flu Season," he states that an unhealthy metabolism limits our cells' ability to return from an excited active state to a calm resting state.[6] This creates long-term, systemic inflammation and emits signals that the cells need to repair.

---

6   Peat, Dr. Ray. "This Novel Flu Season." Ray Peat Forum, June 21, 2020. https://raypeatfo-rum.com/community/threads/ray-peats-newsletter-this-novel-flu-season-may-2020.34831/.

That's what inflammation really is. Ray says pre-existing inflammation is associated with the ability to get sick from a virus, chronic diseases, and altitude sickness.

What dictates a healthy immunity? A healthy metabolism, which includes normalizing your energy production. You then create energy in your body more efficiently by eating organic, high-quality foods, move to create circulation and build muscle, breathe properly, think healthy thoughts, hydrate with minerals, get quality sleep, and live a beautiful, joyful, creative life.

It's surprising that's all it really takes. Yet we're led to believe something so natural is so difficult to achieve and that we need to fix it by adding in things we may not even need and that may even make us sick.

Optimal immune response also requires you to reduce long-term cellular excitation and inflammation. If our immune system is working optimally, the inflammation will activate your adaptive exosome system, which involves converting RNA you get from a virus back into DNA, a process called retrotransposon.[7]

According to the article, "What Are Exosomes," exosomes are defined as small cells that transfer DNA, RNA, and proteins to other cells, which alters the function of target cells that a virus may be going after.[8] For years, they were thought to be transporters of cellu-

7 "Retrotransposon," Wikipedia, last modified September 20, 2021, https://en.wikipedia.org/wiki/Retrotransposon.

8 Cade Hildreth, "What Are Exosomes, Exactly?" *BioInformant*, May 12, 2021, https://bioinformant.com/what-are-exosomes.

lar waste, but there have been recent discoveries that they also play a role in intracellular communication and transportation.

Exosomes are present in nearly all bodily fluids, like your blood, urine, synovial fluid (sacs of fluid around your joints), amniotic fluid, semen, vaginal fluid, breast milk, and much more.

It's truly incredible what the human body is capable of doing. Your immune system has the ability to protect your DNA and overlap the virus production mechanism, says Dr. Ray Peat. When it's working optimally, it's adaptive and creative.

What that science bomb I just dropped on you means is that your cells have the ability to communicate, adapt, and eliminate any harmful toxins or pathogens. This is your body's natural state and what you were born to do.

This is why I stress how important it is to learn how to trust your body and how it handles life. When you take care of your body, you reap the benefits of what it has to offer you.

When we don't take care of our body or we lose our trust in its ability to function well, it responds to us by creating inflammation. There's a signal that something needs to be repaired. Whether it's through anxiety, worry, or fear, these are all equally as destructive to your immune system and create excitatory cells that will not calm down.

When this happens, your cells lose their ability to function properly, and then they can't respond to a virus as previously described through your adaptive immunity. Mainly because the inflammation never gets turned off, so your cells never calm down and get to a resting state. This is what long-term, systemic inflammation does to your body.

Other causes of this systemic inflammation can be eating foods high in polyunsaturated fatty acids like canola oil and soybean oil, which are in just about all processed foods today. If you read your labels, you'll begin to realize how big this issue is and why so many people are susceptible to it.

Not to mention genetically modified foods, which create inflammation in the pests they are trying to kill. When you eat foods that are GMO-based, you get that inflammation in your body over time too. It's systemic, so it's harder to notice because it creeps up over time. Then all of a sudden, you're faced with an autoimmune issue, bewildered as to where it came from.

I say all of this not to scare you or stress you out but instead to bring awareness to what we could change about our daily lives that could impact our health greatly and return our sense of trust in our body again.

It's all about your ability to shut off your inflammation and bring your cells back to a calm resting state. This is what sets you apart from someone who gets sick or suffers from disease and someone who's resilient to it. That's not to say you may never get sick. You most certainly will at times, but how you handle it is what's key.

The difference in a healthy body is that you may not be sick for very long and may not suffer any recurring symptoms afterward. By getting sick and exposing yourself to a virus, you build natural immunity to it, and it makes you stronger. This is what we've always known.

That's what herd immunity is all about. The healthy, younger people get exposed and build immunity to a virus so that it weakens the strength of the virus. This, in some sense, naturally protects the vulnerable people in the herd.

It wasn't until I had a personal experience with my son, who was eighteen months old at the time, where he had a bad reaction to a vaccine that included seizures, severe vomiting, and diarrhea the day he received one of his routine vaccines, that I truly understood this. I sat there and watched as my son went vacant, and I panicked. As traumatizing as it was, it woke me up big time to some of the things that had been going on in both the medical industry and with the CDC. The doctors were telling me that it wasn't the vaccine, yet the side effects listed on the fact sheet they shared with me explained these symptoms were possible in 1 out of every 14,000 recipients of this vaccine. My husband and I were bewildered as to why the doctors would deny this was the case because it seemed so obvious to us. We talked to the nurse, and she told us it was the vaccine and that the doctors are obligated to say that it was not the vaccine to everyone. We could not believe what we had just heard. I felt betrayed and angry that something like this could even happen.

This monumental moment with my son, as scary as it was, led me to learn how to become my own authority in my health.

I wanted to find out more. I wanted to know how the body really worked. So I began my journey of getting curious about the biochemistry of the immune system and how it relates to our current state of health. This led me back to the metabolism, as I mentioned at the beginning of this chapter. I realized that our immune systems are dynamic, just like everything else in nature.

If there's any doubt about something, I always revert back to nature and ask myself, *What would nature do?* My first thought was that our body is a part of nature, so why wouldn't we work like nature? Nothing in nature works separately from itself; it works symbiotically. Why would we expect anything different when it comes to our bodies?

Have you ever planted a garden and noticed how each component depends on the other to grow your food? Nothing separates itself; everything involved has a direct purpose and plays a part in the end result. For example, I planted blueberry bushes one year and waited over two years for any blueberries to come out. I couldn't figure out where I went wrong.

It wasn't until I planted flowers around the blueberries that they started to produce blueberries. I was ecstatic. I couldn't believe I missed that simple fix. Of course, the flowers bring in the insects and the birds to pollinate the blueberry bushes too.

This is incredibly powerful and translates to just about anything we do in our lives, especially as it relates to our creativity and our potential. If you cannot believe in your own body's potential to be creative, how do you expect to believe in yourself?

ACTION STEPS

It all starts with your body and your beliefs. Where do you stand with this? Are you willing to look at a different perspective and open yourself up to new possibilities as it relates to your body?

Check in with these six foundational principles of health: hydration, nutrition, movement, breathing, thoughts, and sleep. Notice if any of these need more attention in your life. Write these down and regularly check in with them.

Six Foundational Health Principles

1. **Hydration:** Drink filtered or mineral-rich spring water, fresh fruit juices, citrus added to water, coconut water, broth, or milk. Are you hydrating often enough?

2. **Nutrition:** Are you eating organic, delicious, and nutritious whole foods to support proper blood sugar regulation?

3. **Movement:** Do you include movement for circulation, mobility, and muscle building daily or weekly?

4. **Breathing:** Are you breathing slow and low and nose breathing during rest and light exercise?

5. **Thoughts:** Are your thoughts adding value to your life and working for you instead of against you?

6. **Sleep:** Are you getting enough sleep to recover physically and mentally from your lifestyle?

CHAPTER 28

YOUR MOOD
AND YOUR FOOD

To some extent, this is how I see us treating our bodies and our appetite. We are taught to override our innate sense of hunger and wait until we are practically binging at our next meal right before we want to bite someone's head off for looking at us wrong.

This is what I mean by *hangry*. Why not instead give your body what it needs by paying attention to it? Starting here is key.

For some people, including myself, our food patterns can reflect how we grew up and what we learned about eating, as well as a traumatic event in our life. If you want to create a new pattern, you have to first become aware of the old pattern when it arises and notice what it looks like and feels like.

In this case, you most likely will fall back into the old pattern once you're stressed, but the good news is that if you can learn how to become aware of the old pattern, you can begin to switch it for a healthier, more desirable pattern once it crops up.

When I was a kid, I'd eat a little bit in the morning, eat an early lunch at school, and then I wouldn't eat for another five hours until I got home from school. Ravenous, I'd binge and head to a four-hour-long gymnastics practice every week day, and then I'd eat ravenously again when I got home around eight or nine in the evening.

Now, my parents didn't intend for me to develop some kind of weird eating pattern like that, but if I was going to be a successful gymnast, that was the sacrifice I had to make at the time. As a result, I go back to this low blood sugar and binge state on occasion. Usually when I'm stressed emotionally, I lose my appetite.

But the good news is that I can use this awareness to broaden my horizon of behaviors around food. Instead of falling into this old pattern permanently, it becomes temporary, and I then move toward new patterns of enjoying my food and eating high-quality, delicious foods. I may make my meal more of an experience and savor it instead of rushing through it.

When I shop for my food, I may talk to local farmers at the farmers' market and buy something I'd not normally cook with. I remind myself of the beauty in food and the experience and feeling of it all.

Seasonal eating is also a real favorite of mine. It breaks up the monotony of eating the same foods over and over, and it's healthier for both your body and the Earth to do so. Eating seasonally means eating differently depending on what the season has to offer and what naturally grows in your region during that time of year.

I also have different go-to foods and food strategies depending on the time of year and the regular nutrient deficiency I'd encounter during that time. This is based on the foods I have access to, outside temperatures, and my amount of sun exposure and time spent inside.

The supplements I implement in the winter are more environmental, like light therapy via infrared sauna, a vitamin D light, dry sauna, and Epsom salt baths. I'm changing my environment, so I'm better able to support both my thyroid and metabolism in more environmentally stressful times.

Since your thyroid is your master regulator of your metabolism, what's good for the thyroid is good for the metabolism. A healthy metabolism is essential for good immune function and more energy. It's all connected.

I'll also add that a healthy disposition is linked to our nutrients. You can wake up in a funk every morning and not even realize you may be missing something as important as vitamin A and copper in your diet, which could be a game-changer for your mood.

This could be one reason we have seasonal depression—the lack of nutrients that are available in the winter as opposed to the sunny summertime. Dark days without proper nutrients and light can be a recipe for depression and fatigue if we aren't paying attention.

Remedy this by paying attention to what your nutrient needs are in each season. Include shellfish in your diet, which is a wonderful source of both vitamin A and copper. Organ meats like liver and kidney are rich sources of vitamin A too. Adding these foods in the wintertime can make all the difference in your health and well-being since these nutrients tend to be lower in most people this time of year.

ACTION STEP

Reflect on your personal food patterns. How do you eat when you are under stress?

Bring awareness to this pattern by identifying it and then changing it in the moment. How can you support yourself when you are stressed? What feels nurturing and healthy?

CHAPTER 29

LIGHTEN YOUR TOXIC LOAD

THE MOST POWERFUL BEAUTY SECRET I HAVE TO SHARE IS something that sounds decidedly un-pretty: toxic load. I've always believed less is more. I've never been one to be attached to beauty products, but I know so many women are. And this is okay; if something works, it works.

Many skin-care and makeup products are filled with toxins that can overstress the body, causing all kinds of unwanted side effects such as dry skin and aging. Remember what I said about rest and recovery earlier? If our bodies are taxed from having to sift through and filter out a heavy toxic load, it won't be resting or regenerating the way it's meant to, which can lead to all manner of chronic wellness problems. I'll add here that toxic body-care products play a role in slowing down your liver's ability to function well. Since your liver is your main detoxification organ, it is important to understand the toxic load of anything you're digesting—through your food *and* skin. The more toxins in, the slower your liver becomes.

And since much of your hormonal conversion happens in the liver, it's equally as important to realize the part your liver plays in looking more youthful.

Again, less is more. The less work you give your liver in the way of toxins, the more energy your liver will have to divert to converting your thyroid and youth steroid hormones that are anti-inflammatory. You'll have clearer, more youthful skin because of it, and your cells will regenerate at a faster pace by keeping your beauty products simple and toxin-free.

Take a look in your bathroom cabinets. How many products do you own and use that have a high toxic load, like parabens that extend shelf life, fragrances, foaming agents like sodium sulfate, artificial colors like Red 40 or Yellow 6, petroleum in the form of mineral oil, formaldehyde used to prevent bacterial growth but also to embalm people, phthalates used in nail polish that are used to soften plastics and are endocrine disruptors, preservatives like BHA or BHT, antibacterial agents, dibutyl phthalate used to harden the product in nail polish, siloxanes that create that smoothness, and thickening agents like PEG compounds, to name a few. You are putting at least twelve, if not more, major chemicals on and in your body when you use these products. What this does to our endocrine systems is unfathomable if we use a lot of them. That's why letting many, if not all, of these products go can be one of the easiest and best things you can do for your health right off the bat.[9]

9 Katie Wells, "10 Toxic Ingredients to Avoid in Personal Care Products," *Wellness Mama, May 12, 2020,* https://wellnessmama.com/426233/toxic-ingredients.

ACTION STEP

Are you willing to let these go and buy products that have a lower toxic load?

Read the labels on your skincare products and makeup. If there's a high toxic load, consider changing these products out for a less toxic organic version.

CHAPTER 30

THE VALUE OF TAKING ACTION

HOLDING YOURSELF ACCOUNTABLE BY TAKING CONSISTENT action is the only way you'll find out if something is working or not. It reinforces your beliefs about yourself and what you are truly capable of, and it creates a relationship of trust, devotion, and confidence with your body.

This is powerful stuff.

This is not about doing more for the sake of doing. It's about the act of showing up for yourself consistently that gives you a sense of self-worth, purpose, and a clear idea of what is working for you. Taking conscious action is a great way to build trust in yourself.

The more we can trust our body's abilities, the better we're able to support it in a way that leads to more energy, better health, and more happiness.

The question is: is it consistent action and focus that gets us where we want to go, or is it an actual change in our core beliefs as we go through the process?

For example, if I wanted to lose weight, I'd start by tracking my food, learning how to eat better, and starting a consistent movement practice. Would I lose weight because of those steps, or because of my belief in myself and my focus on how I was directing my body?

Because of this process of taking action and focus, I now have more confidence, trust, and self-worth. I can feel how good it is to take care of myself without shame or blame. It's probably a little bit of everything, but nonetheless, this is powerful stuff.

I know losing weight can be a real trigger for many people, and I think that's mainly due to the emotional charge that so many people have around it. I use this as an example because it all relates back to perspective. If your belief lies in whether you can lose weight or not, it'll happen that way. If you have emotional trauma or blocks around this, it will inhibit your progress.

The act of consistent action will build your confidence to do this over time as well as allow you to see your blocks and emotional triggers, and to clear them or allow them to move through in the process. That's why it's important to give yourself a real opportunity to have a process.

Whether someone loses weight or reaches their goal because of a perspective change or because of how they are eating or moving, I don't really know. What I do know is that when a person starts taking action, they start to feel good, and they begin to heal on a deeper level by providing the space, time, and attention for consistent action.

By taking this consistent action, you are communicating to your body that it matters to you and that you value it because you are devoting that time and attention to your body. Your body will respond with health and well-being, which will reflect the love you are giving it.

You then have changed a belief about yourself just by taking inspired action.

ACTION STEP

What are you wanting to do? What are three inspired action steps you can take right now? Write these down, and then begin implementing them today.

PART III

LISTEN TO
YOUR SPIRIT

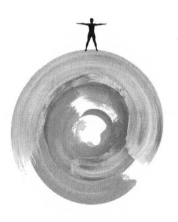

CHAPTER 31

YOU ARE A CONSCIOUS CREATOR OF YOUR BODY

"The physical world, including our bodies, is a response of the observer. We create our bodies as we create the experience of our world."

—Deepak Chopra

YOUR CELLS ARE REGENERATING THEMSELVES CONSTANTLY, building a new body every seven years. If this is true, then what we think about ourselves is important because this will give your body direction on what to build on a cellular level. How you perceive yourself and your life will shape how you experience it.

In her book, *Buddhist Mandalas: Explore Parallel Realities with Sacred Geometry,* Von Galt describes how we can jump from reality to reality based upon our perception of ourselves.

She also mentions that energy is more real than anything else, and I tend to agree. Our energy is the only thing that we can take with us when we leave this earthly plane. What's even more fascinating is that we have what she describes as "energy signatures," which reflect our unique ways of consciously creating our reality.

I love this way of seeing ourselves.

If this is true, why aren't all of our health dreams coming to fruition as soon as we think about them?

Most of us are still trapped in a perspective of duality. This or that. Good or bad. Black or white. Them or me. But actually, many things can be true, all at once.

For example, if we're always in a state of stress, we'll age faster. Stress comes in many forms, but for a majority of us, it's a product of fear that typically arises out of harsh self-criticism.

We're our own worst critics. We're so hard on ourselves, and most of the time, other people don't even notice what we're seeing wrong within ourselves. What we fail to realize is that other people don't pay attention to or judge us nearly as much as we judge ourselves. The truth is, most people probably don't even notice.

Perfectionism could be part of it. It was definitely that for me. While perfectionism can be extremely limiting and restrictive, it also doesn't allow you to play, since messing up or being really vulnerable would mean that you're not perfect.

No, you're not perfect, you're human. And humans are vulnerable. They connect and they mess up, but they also put themselves out there, take chances, and find joy in the process. That's living.

Learning how you play is important for knowing yourself enough to know what motivates you and for discovering your passion. Plus, everything we learn in life starts from a point of imperfection.

Your own inner critic can stop you in your tracks before you get started if you let it. In my experience, it's about the fear of judgment. What will other people think if I stand out or do something different?

In my case, this was a feeling first brought on by my experiences in elementary school. When I was young, the culture was not supportive of children like it is now, so what I experienced felt pretty traumatizing. I was a very active kid who could barely sit still, and I had ADHD. Luckily, I did not have to take medication for the ADHD because gymnastics was a great remedy for it, but I was taking allergy medicine that was the equivalent of speed. So, needless to say, I got in trouble often with my teachers.

I hated school, which was unfortunate because I remember being so excited initially about going to school and the potential of making new friends and learning new things. I remember thinking how much fun kindergarten was, but when I got to first grade, everything changed.

Sitting in a chair all day was miserable. I could no longer play, and I had a teacher that was not supportive and downright mean to me on a daily basis. I'd get in trouble constantly for talking and getting up out of my chair. I thought to myself: *What is this? This isn't what I thought it would be.* Before long, I started to feel like I was getting in trouble for being me.

Now, as an adult, I understand how disruptive that can be for a teacher, but as a first grader, I took that experience to heart. How ridiculous is it to make kids sit down all day?

Later, around sixth grade, I was constantly bullied by a boy at my school, and my teachers weren't very supportive or loving. This experience left me feeling very defensive. I felt like everyone was against me, and at the age of twelve, I began to get extremely depressed, feeling very alone.

I thought to myself, I'd better change who I am because "who I am" is pissing people off, so I'd better become someone they could like. So that's what I did, I became a person that would fit into any situation—a shapeshifter, if you will. I did my best to avoid conflict and to never rock the boat.

When I reflect on it, I realize I put a ton of unrealistic pressure on myself to be perfect in the eyes of others, never letting them see the real me in the hopes that I'd never risk feeling that kind of pain again.

I appreciate how essential it was for me to respond that way because otherwise, I don't know if, at that age, I could have taken much more. I'm truly grateful for my twelve-year-old for doing what she needed to survive. The problem is, it doesn't serve me anymore, and I dare say it's even stifling me at this point in my life.

A friend of mine once described it like this: You wore pants when you were younger that fit you, but you wouldn't try to keep wearing those pants now because you've grown out of them. The same goes for your emotional responses and how you perceived the world when you were younger. As you grow, they change. It's about the awareness of whether we're still trying to fit into those small pants.

There's so much stress and pressure in dimming yourself to fit in. It can be downright depleting never letting other people see the real you. I'd quite honestly done it for so long I couldn't even remember who the real Allison was anymore.

I share this about myself because as children in our formative years, we take our experiences to heart. It's important to understand this about yourself because this is what shapes our reality as adults and how we respond to life. You may think a painful childhood memory is not that important to your daily adult life, but until you resolve it, this story will keep running in the background. Then you're left feeling blocked or can't figure out why you're in a particular behavioral pattern.

I had to go through a process of rediscovering myself so that I could be a more honest, less judgmental, more creative, and joyful person. I learned how to expose myself and allowed other people to take responsibility for how they experience me.

I also accept the consequences of being myself, whatever those may be. Not to mention how this greatly benefited my health by taking a huge burden of stress off my shoulders.

ACTION STEP

What in your life triggered you to dim to fit in? If you were free to be you, what would your life look like? Can you accept where you are right now by loving yourself enough to want to make a change for the better?

It takes trust in oneself and courage to see it through.

CHAPTER 32

ARE YOU DISTRACTING YOURSELF FROM YOURSELF?

OFTENTIMES WHEN HEALTH ISSUES COME UP, WE THINK THE solution to solving our health puzzle is to treat the diagnosis. This is like putting a bandage on a deep wound. It's surface area healing instead of really getting to the root of the issue. That's okay at first because many times, the trauma is so deep that we may not be ready to get to the root of it, but keep in mind, it's not a long-term solution.

Going from practitioner to practitioner is not the answer either. You start to look at your problem only from a physical perspective, even if you're approaching it from a functional medicine standpoint. I see it all of the time; tons of supplements are prescribed along with a massively impossible protocol.

This just loads you with more stress. Change is stressful enough, so the last thing people need is more to-do items loaded on their plate. The people I work with most often need less.

Why are people making it harder on themselves?

I think it's a way we learn how to distract ourselves from ourselves. It's hard to be with yourself, and for many people, it's much easier to get on social media, watch Netflix, or get caught up in their work or the drama of the day. It makes sense that we'd want to distract ourselves even more by adding more distractions. We work until we're so exhausted that the strategy of distraction just won't work anymore.

I'm not saying all these physical approaches are not helpful. Heck, I spend most of my time teaching my clients how to navigate the physical, and I talk about many in this book. It's extremely necessary, but if you are doing many physical actions and not resolving the issue, I invite you to begin to look at it a different way.

Weigh the level of stress in your life first before you go forward piling a bunch of to-do items that are in addition to the other to-do items you already have in your life. This will not help you, and oftentimes, it'll make things worse.

For example, over-burdening the liver with more supplements when you already have a very hard time digesting your food is not a good idea. It's like putting extra weight on a body that's already struggling.

Instead, we need to lift some burdens to aid in the healing process, physically and energetically allowing space to move into a new way of being. You probably wouldn't buy more clothes if your closet was stuffed to the brim. You'd most likely get rid of the clothes you don't wear anymore to make space for the new clothes you want to buy and wear.

The same goes for your health. You must make space for a new energy embodiment so that you can make changes and then integrate them into your lifestyle.

Making a drastic change that is just not enjoyable with your food and lifestyle is not necessary and, quite frankly, makes people more adverse to making positive changes in their health. It makes it seem really hard to get healthy when that's not the case at all. For so many of us, it can be simple, fun, and easy if we want it to be.

I invite you to buy in fully to the change that you're making in order for it to stick because change is hard enough; you might as well enjoy it. Feeling uncomfortable is normal when you're going through change because what you're creating is the body of art that is your life.

You are learning new skills and then implementing them. This takes more energy, time, and persistence, as you are ultimately learning how to give yourself the time, love, and attention you need to thrive. Get to the heart of what needs to be healed so that you can create what you want in your life.

Come up with a plan that you can live with, one that's not so extreme and one that you enjoy exploring with a childlike curiosity. A plan that you can truly integrate into your life and that speaks to your heart. A plan that brings all the parts of yourself together as a whole.

ACTION STEP

How can you make yourself a priority each day? Start by taking one hour to be with yourself. Whether it's a workout, a walk, journaling, a float tank session, yoga, meditation. This time is precious, and it teaches you the value of spending time with yourself. Nobody matters most to you but you.

Go back to the examples I gave for a wellness date and have daily wellness dates with yourself. Honoring your body and health is the best investment you can make in your time and energy. Learning how to be present with yourself allows you to become present with others and value your time with them.

CHAPTER 33

LIVING IN REVERENCE

Living in reverence is to respect ourselves and others by honoring ourselves.

Are you in alignment with your personal standards? Are you changing those standards as you grow? Do you know what you will and won't tolerate in your relationships?

These are important questions to explore. If you aren't aware of these, it's impossible to go into any situation with any sense of where you begin and where others end, as well as what you'll put up with.

So many times I've justified or ridiculed other people's behaviors in the hopes of a situation working out in my favor. In other words, I'd compromise my own standard to make other people happy, also known as people-pleasing, only to realize that I wasn't taking responsibility for my own life because I wasn't being honest about my personal standards.

The truth is, we as individuals can set standards for ourselves and get clear about what we do or do not wish to tolerate in our lives. This becomes extremely empowering because you can't change what others do, but you can decide what you want for yourself.

This allows other people to then decide if they want to be a part of that. You become more trustable in a relationship because now you are being honest about how you feel and what's important to you.

This was hard for me at first because I'd been taught to fix things in relationships. To avoid hurting my partner's feelings or to feel like I needed to make everything better. What I discovered was that people-pleasing left me feeling like I was in a codependent relationship. Codependent on what I perceived as my partner's perception instead of exploring my own happiness, only to find myself more confused, not truly knowing how to express and communicate my needs to my partner.

This also left my partner feeling unsure if I was being honest or just trying to please him. He needed to know what my wants, desires, and needs were so that he could trust me.

Intimacy starts with yourself. If you cannot be intimate with yourself by acknowledging your desires, then it's impossible for a partner to do it. If you want to have a better relationship with other people, start by exploring your own wants first.

We often suppress our desires and wants, and then when we see other people playing those desires out, we negatively project our fears onto them or beat ourselves up.

Why not stop projecting and start reflecting? When we can reflect on a possible unmet desire within ourselves, we're less triggered when we see other people playing it out. Instead, we are cheering them on because we can now see ourselves in them.

I see it like this: Your true desires are telling you what you are here to do. They are a clue to your direction in life. They will lead you exactly where you want to go and what you want to create. We get a sense of this when we are children. We are drawn to certain things because we are curious to learn more about them. These are clues as to what your purpose here is and could potentially become.

What I mean by true desire is not what you learned from other people or society about what you should want. True desires are more of what comes from within. You most likely had these same desires when you were a kid, but somewhere along the way, you started to suppress these desires as you became an adult. It's actually more of a feeling and an experience than a material thing.

How do we connect with those desires again?

The best way to start acknowledging your desires is to see what's there by writing some down. It can be anything from buying a new sofa to getting a new piece of art on the wall to painting the art yourself. What are you wanting to do that you aren't doing? What are you stopping yourself from doing for fear you'll get what you want?

My teacher Paul Chek would say, "What you resist persists."

What this means to me is that the more we suppress our desires, the more the shadow side of that desire comes up in our lives. So, for example, if you want to be wealthy but you have a story you tell yourself about wealthy people being greedy and bad, you will continue to experience the shadow side of wealth. This is a scarcity mentality.

This goes the same with your body. If you are always creating a story about people who look good on Instagram, for example, but you secretly wish you could look like that or do the things they are doing, you will always experience the shadow side of expression, which is not feeling like you are enough, making yourself small, or having a victim mentality.

ACTION STEP

Your practice here is to acknowledge what you want by making a list of what you will not tolerate anymore and then making another list of what you desire. Don't hold back; anything goes.

CHAPTER 34

YOUR MULTIDIMENSIONAL SELF

"There are no victims here, only masters."

—Rosanne Grace

DID YOU KNOW THAT YOU ACTUALLY HAVE TWO BODIES? WELL, really, a lot more than that, but for the sake of simplicity, we'll call it two. Your physical body and your subtle energy body. Your physical body allows you to feel, see, and experience your energy on this physical plane. It's your vehicle, so to speak. Your physical body responds and adapts to your subtle energy body.

Your subtle energy body is actually more you. It reflects reality in a way that crosses all time and space. It's your essence, and it will show you the way. It's your intuition, your higher self, your inner child, and your future self. It's your multidimensional self.

When we talk about 5D wellness, learning to connect to your subtle body is key. We all go through stages in our health and wellness, but in the fifth dimension, we're bridging the gap heavily between the energetic and the physical body.

Before we get into 5D, let me explain a little about what 3D and 4D wellness represent. In 3D, we're learning about the physical. How it all works, your body and its processes, and the right way to exercise and eat. All the structural components of health. Essentially, your framework.

It's okay if you're here; you're in the right place. This can even be about the quality of food and the integrity around regenerative farming and the kind of food companies you'd like to support with your dollars. Your basic foundation.

Meanwhile, 4D is more in the realm of embodiment. How you bring the information into your body and integrate it and begin to practice it. It's the process of learning how to feel and connect with the changes in your body on an emotional level. Learning how to navigate your emotional body and your physical body and the interplay between the two.

Through movement, you begin to release emotions or evoke strength and stability. It's the next level of awareness in your health journey.

Our 5D self is all about strengthening your awareness of your subtle energetic body and connecting it with your physical body. They work together, and believe it or not, your physical body is able to change and shift according to your energetic body. 5D wellness is about bringing the practice of intention into your experience, only you must experience the other levels first.

The term spiritual bypassing best describes trying to jump to the next level without mastering the one before it first. Although you can certainly try to go straight to the fifth dimension, you'll have to eventually learn how to navigate the body by keeping it healthy and learning how to navigate your emotions first. This is what grounds you into this physical reality. Otherwise, you won't get very far on this physical plane because you must learn how to ground yourself if you want to experience your energy in an empowered way.

In 5D, your desires manifest much quicker because you're connecting with them on a deeper level. You're feeling the changes and changing your beliefs about yourself. You're able to change your body on a cellular level with intention. This work goes deep.

You have more energy, and it's easy and fun to maintain your health because you enjoy your practice. You own your practice wholeheartedly because you're not doing it for anyone but the love of yourself. This love spills out to everyone you come across.

You're able to open up to your subtle energetic body and navigate it in a way that serves you, in a way that is more discerning to your energy output and where you'd like to focus. You have a deep knowledge about what your body needs and trust that your body knows what to do to keep you healthy and safe.

You realize that this body is malleable and that you are able to feel as youthful as you'd like because you know how to recover, regenerate, and visualize. You treat your body like the fine-tuned machine it is and navigate it with great reverence. This is leveling up, my friend.

I never understood this as much as I do now, all due to the work I've done with my incredible mentors and teachers. My coach, Hanna Bier, in particular, has taught me how to harness my energy and live life with the intention of becoming the architect of my life. Rosanne Grace has taught me how to connect with my inner child like no one else has before. Both of these women have taught me the skills to become my own guru, my own guide, and to connect with my soul.

This has been a lifelong search for answers. I've worked with countless healers and coaches. I've participated in many work-shops, coaching intensives, and energy work classes over the years. I've also studied a plethora of different spiritual philosophies over this time, but not one has brought me to learn how to play. You see, I discovered that play is the most spiritual experience there is because it leads to joy and bliss. Joy and bliss are two of the highest forms of love.

I'll admit that could have just been me not seeing it. Maybe there were some teachings in there about cultivating play, fun, and joy, but I don't recall any such thing. I could chalk it up to not being open to it at the time. I may have needed to experience the suffering first.

Now, I wouldn't trade my journey for anything, and I feel that it was all necessary for my growth. Looking back on it, I realized it was missing one major component: fun. I hadn't realized that I was taking the joy out of the process by taking life too seriously.

I always thought I needed to suffer to find my purpose and to level up my consciousness. Lucky for me, I started working with two incredible coaches who taught me some simple and very effective concepts that blew me away. It suddenly became so much easier to connect my physical and energetic bodies and see amazing manifestations and synchronicities because of it.

I never really put it together until I realized that what I was feeling was real and that much of it was my energetic body trying to communicate to me through my physical body.

You see, we all have different ways of connecting with our intuition. Mainly through acknowledging, practicing, and developing these gifts. We all have this connection in some form or another, and we can develop, practice, and strengthen our intuition just like developing a skill in a sport or for your job. By practicing these skills over time, your energy begins working for you instead of against you. You learn to become more open, aware, and intentional.

I'm more of what people would call a feeler. I feel what other people are feeling. When I was younger, it was challenging because I didn't really know what to do with the information. I could pick up on someone's energy really easily, and then I'd say something to my parents and be embarrassed or feel ashamed because it could come off kind of rude, and then I'd get in trouble. As a child, I'd just know if someone had ill intentions, and I'd speak out about it.

The responses I'd get from my parents were confusing. I understand now that being a parent is a balancing act, and as a kid, you take the response you get from your parents to heart. In your formative years, this shapes you, who you become, and how you respond to the world as an adult.

So although my parents had the best of intentions by teaching me how to be a part of our community while being respectful to others, I still walked away feeling like I'd done something wrong. This felt like it was a part of me that people did not like.

As I grew from a child to an adult, I tried to ignore these feelings that I'd picked up about other people and even took other people's feelings as my own. Until one day, I didn't know where I stopped and others began.

Of course, becoming a trainer and teaching people about health and exercise ended up being a perfect profession for me. It allowed me to channel that information into helping people help themselves.

I realized I never got any instruction on how to navigate my energetic body. I wondered for years if it was real. I thought it was only my imagination, that it wasn't really happening. Only to realize that, yes, it's real and it's my imagination, and yes, my imagination is real too.

Once I acknowledged that within myself, my life took a turn for the better. Instead of feeling separate from my subtle energy body, I finally felt connected to it like I never had before.

It was as if after all these years, it was confirmed that, Allison, no, you were not a silly child with crazy ideas. You actually nailed it. You were right all along; you just didn't have anyone who could teach you that.

ACTION STEPS

How do you acknowledge this within yourself? You ground yourself in the 3D with proper food, movement, and sleep practices. You connect yourself in the 4D by learning how to navigate your emotional body. Let your emotions move through as you learn how to observe them.

Then you integrate yourself in the 5D by bringing your subtle energy body in the mix and learning how to feel your subtle energy body with discernment in the physical body.

You become your own guru.

The practice here is to follow your intuition. Once you get calm and grounded in your body, you can begin to practice trusting yourself. Even if something doesn't make sense at that moment but feels right, go with it and see where it takes you. For example, you get an intuitive hit to take a different route to work one morning or you have an urge to call a certain friend or you are called to pick up a certain book. These are all subtle ways you can begin to trust your intuition.

Even just making decisions and paying attention to the outcome is a start. Whether it serves you or not is a way we can begin to learn how to trust ourselves. I used to beat myself up if I made a so-called wrong decision, but now I realize that it's just part of the process of learning how to trust your intuition. It's feedback, and you are getting to decide what you want to create too.

Developing your intuitive abilities and trusting yourself is a practice you do and test out every day. From my experience, this can be very serendipitous. Bring your awareness to what you might not normally notice in your life. This is how you become your own guru.

CHAPTER 35

ENERGY IN MOTION

"Dance like no one is watching because they're not. They're all checking their cell phones."

—Unknown

YOU ARE ENERGY IN MOTION. IF YOU WERE TO STOP MOVING completely at your most basic expression of movement, which is breathing, you'd be dead. Even if you sit at a desk all day long without moving, you're still energy in motion.

According to the book, *Back to a Future for Mankind, Biogeometry,* by Ibrahim Karim, energy is measured by quality rather than quantity. In fact, biogeometry is the science of quality, as Ibrahim describes. This is one reason I think the scientific community does not address many things that relate to energy in the esoteric realm. It's almost impossible to measure the quality of something that is experiential, like an energy signature.

We all have what I call a movement signature. A way you move that is unique only to you. Much like your voice signature, you express this in your everyday movement too. Only things like restrictive clothes, shoes, and chairs can get in the way of how we were born to move.

When you develop as a young child from infant to toddler, you're creating your signature moves. What's fascinating is that there's no mistake in what we go through in the way of infant development as we're learning how to lift our heads, sit up, roll over, and eventually stand and walk. It's incredible if you're able to witness this phenomenon.

If we're born with an innate knowledge of how to move, then why do we seem to lose some of those abilities as we get older?

Blame it on our lifestyle of sitting at a desk all day, staring at a computer, or just vegging out in front of the television. It all plays a part. I'd also dare say that the way we dress and express ourselves plays a part too. Well, this is how functional and natural movement training came to be. There was a need to help people get back to the basics and learn how to move again instinctively.

When's the last time you danced like no one was watching? Did you move without thinking about it, despite feeling silly? Kids demonstrate this all the time. I remember being enamored by my son when he was younger, when he'd dance and move his body at the drop of a hat. We'd walk by a street performer, and he would stop and just break into dance. He'd move to the energy of the music, and it was so joyful to watch. I'd think to myself, *I wish I could be that uninhibited. What a beautiful way to be.*

Of course, judgment from others gets in the way too. Judgment affects our movement signature directly, inhibiting it. How many of us need a few drinks to get on the dance floor? How many of us can dance at the drop of a hat in the grocery store when we hear a good song? How many people hold back? I've always thought it'd be so much fun if everyone in the grocery store just broke out into dance, and we all just had this moment together and then went about our day.

How fun would that be? Yet we don't do that, and what happens as a result trains us to hold back on our movement a little more each day until, one day, we have nothing. No connection whatsoever to our personal movement signature.

One thing I offer to my clients is to dance at home like no one's watching. Turn on your favorite song and just move your body to the music without thinking about it. Allow your body to move intuitively with the rhythm. This'll allow you to explore different signature moves and work through the feeling of judgment around your movement. You'll get to know what your unique moves feel and look like.

I especially love to do this when I cook. I'll put on some good music and dance to my heart's content. It's truly the most fun thing ever. It's fun when my husband walks in on me when I'm doing this too. Sometimes he'll join in and dance with me.

What comes up for you when you do this? How does it make you feel? Are you having fun with it, or do you feel silly? Is it painful? Whatever comes up is totally okay. It's a normal part of the process of peeling the layers so you can get to your true essence.

This practice will surprisingly translate into your life and how you express yourself in the world. You'll no longer have to think about how you'll show up in the world; you'll just show up as you are, and it'll be easy. You may find that you're no longer hiding parts of yourself from others. It's so subtle yet incredibly powerful.

We'll usually hide parts of ourselves to fit in, and if you think about it, it definitely makes a person less trustworthy to others when they're constantly holding parts of themself back. Hiding parts of ourselves to fit in also depletes our energy over time.

This practice will help you get to know yourself better in this way. Movement is also a way we communicate with others. It's a language and a form of personal expression. You can move and sometimes communicate more to someone than if you were to speak.

For example, children, before they know how to talk, have the ability to communicate without words. You know right away if they're upset, hungry, or tired without them even having to say a word. They may drop to the floor and cry or make a face.

Yet we use so many words to explain how we feel. Ironically, this takes the feeling right out of it and brings us into more of a headspace.

Another way to connect with your movement signature is to pay attention first to what feelings come up as you move in certain ways. How can you allow these feelings to move through in that moment?

I've been in sessions with clients where we're just doing a simple hip lift on a Swiss ball, and they just start crying. They're instantly bewildered as to why they're crying for no perceived reason, but I explain that movement can move emotions through that are being held in the body. This is truly a gift.

Expressing our feelings through movement can be incredibly healing. Allow your emotions to move through without judgment. Your Chakras can be activated by certain key movements, which allow you to connect to what is out of balance.

Don't use words—just movement. If your partner is into it, you can play a game and just communicate what you're trying to say through your body language. This could be why people love playing Charades. It's an opportunity to get back to our primal nature of communication.

ACTION STEP

Improvisational dancing is the best way to connect to your movement signature.

Start by putting your favorite song on, or one that reflects your current mood, and start dancing. Notice how your body wants to move instead of directing your body to move. Then let your body move however it feels like moving.

Like a choral director channels the energy of their musicians and singers with instruments and voice, you can channel and direct the energies that live in your body this way too.

The first time I did this, it was really uncomfortable because as a gymnast, I was taught to make all of my movements purposeful and beautiful. What I learned was that I had a whole range of moves I hadn't even tapped into yet. Some of them were totally silly and awkward, but those were the most fun. Improv dancing allowed me to expose all the shadows I was hiding from other people, thus dissipating the hold that the worry of looking silly or awkward had over me. I'd never realized how liberating it could be to let myself go in that way before.

Dance while you're cooking or just dance when you feel like it. Notice how this feels in your body. What comes up for you?

CHAPTER 36

RETURN
TO INNOCENCE

INNOCENCE IS THE HIGHEST FORM OF LOVE. BRINGING YOURSELF
back to your childlike innocence by connecting with your inner
child is pure love. This is a concept that's fairly new to many
of us.

We have to connect with our childlike innocence and curiosity to
tap into our true essence.

I'm reminded of Baby Yoda when I think about this. The energy
of "The Child," as he's called in the series, is pure innocence that
evokes pure love from others when they are in his presence. You
cannot help but love him and see how powerful he is all at once.
They are one and the same.

For those who have yet to watch *The Mandalorian,* the Mandalorian soldier is charged with protecting The Child and bringing
him to a Jedi who'll be able to train him on how to harness his
powers.

"Baby Yoda" is a representation of pure innocence, our essence. The Mandalorian sees in The Child what is really within himself and becomes devoted to protecting that pure innocence no matter what. He, after all, lost his innocence as a child. He finds it again when he meets The Child. Baby Yoda reminded him that his true innocence lies within him, and he must protect it at any cost.

It is one of the best analogies that I can think of when it comes to connecting with this pure innocence within all of us.

This innocence is in each and every one of us. We all have the ability to tap into this pure innocence anytime we'd like. It's our natural state, and this is ultimately the game to play. If you can see this in yourself, you can begin to see it in others.

It brings an entirely new level of compassion to the mix and a way to bridge the gap between what's blocking us from loving each other, experiencing the beauty of our lives, knowing true bliss, and ultimately loving ourselves. Regaining the innocence within ourselves frees us from our suffering. We are perfect just the way we are.

This hit home for me most when I realized that I denied my childlike innocence around the age of six in an effort to keep my parents together. I took on the energy of taking care of my family instead of being taken care of as a child. Many of us have had this experience. Thinking this is how we can keep our family together or keep others happy.

I thought I could fix it by picking a sport like gymnastics that required my family to spend endless hours driving to practice, going to gymnastics meets every weekend, and even having my whole family volunteer and participate. Heck, I got my family so involved with the sport my sister even made the team, and my dad eventually became a gymnastics judge after he retired. I had my family in deep.

Little did I realize this wasn't gonna work. Despite my valiant efforts, it didn't work, and my family ended up breaking apart. I was left feeling like I'd spent all this time sacrificing, and for what? Nothing.

I didn't realize, until much later, that I'd sacrificed my childhood innocence by pleasing other people. I learned that "people-pleasing" is just another form of manipulation.

I healed by rediscovering my desire to play, create, and explore. I had to learn what it meant to be me and to move toward things that inspired me instead of what I felt obligated to do, so I could do it out of love for myself and my childlike curiosity.

Can you pinpoint when you became self-aware or started to lose your childhood innocence?

This isn't meant to rehash old trauma for you but to bring attention to the awareness around what innocence really means for you.

ACTION STEP

What does innocence mean to you, and how can you connect with it?

Maybe it's an afternoon spent doing nothing or that feeling when you fall in love with someone and you get to explore each other with curiosity and joy. Maybe it's creating something for the sake of creating. Whatever it is, spend some time there today.

When we can connect to our pure innocence, we can begin to see this in other people. We see the inherent beauty within all things. We find joy in our everyday lives, and we begin to slowly reclaim our true selves.

CHAPTER 37

ACKNOWLEDGING TRAUMA

WHEN WE DIMINISH OUR TRAUMA, NO MATTER HOW BIG OR HOW small we perceive it to be, we discount our pain. This leaves us never feeling and transmuting the pain into something more powerful. This affects our bodies.

We lose our ability to feel if we do this too much. I used to diminish my trauma by comparing it to other people's trauma and discounting it because it didn't seem traumatic enough compared to the level of pain another person was experiencing.

This was a mistake because by doing this, I did not allow myself to feel the pain and allow it to move through, thus creating more disconnection in my body.

So many of my clients come in very disconnected from their bodies. This is so common. It's a rare thing to see people who are fully in their bodies.

This is because we naturally disconnect from feeling our pain, either physically or emotionally or both. Until one day, the physical pain becomes so great you cannot ignore it anymore.

This is a consequence of not acknowledging our trauma or how we understood something as children and took it to heart, no matter how big or small we perceive it to be. It all matters.

Once you acknowledge this, you can feel it and move it through.

The other side of the coin is that we can over-identify with our trauma, turning us into a victim who identifies with being pathetic or pitiful. Did you know that being pathetic is just as powerful as being arrogant? They're two sides of the same coin. They're both ways of getting attention when our emotional needs are not being met.

Now I recommend getting with a good coach or therapist to support you through this process because depending on what comes up for you and where you are with it, you may need guidance and someone to hold space for you.

ACTION STEP

Working with a skilled therapist or coach will provide you with a safe, supportive, and trusting environment to release what needs to be released and felt.

CHAPTER 38

CELEBRATE
YOUR WINS

FOR MANY YEARS, I'D GET STUCK IN A PLACE WITH MYSELF OF JUST focusing on fixing what I perceived was wrong with me. My attention was on what needed to heal, what I didn't like about my body, what was painful, what was out of alignment, what was uncomfortable.

Of course, I needed to acknowledge what was happening, but I was making the mistake of doing that without acknowledging what was working. When you only focus on what needs to be fixed until it gets fixed, you can never see what's working. Not to mention it's endless. You have no direction. This "fix it" mentality leaves you feeling constantly anxious about your body because you're in the dark with it. Always looking for the next fix, so to speak.

You suffer because you're constantly struggling to attain something that is unattainable. Could that be why so many people become their problem? They start identifying with their illness or issue, and it becomes who they are.

Then you get into a vicious cycle of your job now becoming these issues you are constantly trying to fix. Why don't we instead take a different path—one of acceptance, love, and taking inspired action? Realize that there is a process and learn how to hold space for it.

As you acknowledge what works along with what needs to be worked on, you begin to see your path. Plus, you develop patience for what your body's process looks and feels like.

Why is this important? It's important because whether you are on a healing journey or just trying to get fit, your body responds to your thinking. If you're always focusing on what's wrong, your body will respond by amplifying what's wrong. It may even give you more things that could go wrong.

Learning how to hold space for my body and all its processes has been one of my most valuable lessons. Since your body responds immediately to what your mind is communicating to it, you must learn how to become more mindful and intentional when it comes to your body.

If you can begin to balance that out with seeing the big picture that is your body and celebrating your wins, you can hold space for recalibration and the process your body must go through to readjust and heal. This will lead to you creating a calmer disposition and becoming the observer and supporter of your body.

It's more of an opening up to an understanding of how your body works and holding space for that. Don't try to rush your body into giving you what you want right away. It'll give you what you want; you just have to focus on what that is and then support it.

For example, when someone is going through a healing process or has an old injury and wants to move more athletically, there are phases that the body must go through to heal that injury. A person must learn how to support the body in its recovery process by learning how to eat, rest, and move for recovery.

If you have an old back injury that keeps cropping up, are you doing the same thing and expecting different results, or are you truly trying something different? Are you making daily stretches a practice? Are you doing hip and core activation before you work out? Are you even learning how to prep your body before you work out?

The question is, are you doing the work, or are you just learning a billion things you could do without integrating it? This is an issue for so many people.

Taking responsibility for yourself sounds kind of boring, I know, but I assure you it's the only way to fly. Because taking responsibility and holding yourself accountable means you are owning your experience. Only then can you become aware of what truly needs to change to tap into unlimited potential.

Taking responsibility and holding yourself accountable is your cornerstone. It's a tool for creating your framework. It means responding with inspired action. Taking consistent inspired action is the best way to discover if something is working or not.

When you discover what works, celebrate it. Celebrating your wins, as little or as big as they are, is paramount. It sends a signal to your body that you are excited about the direction you are going in and to keep the wins coming with directed focus on what works.

ACTION STEP

Write out three of your wins and acknowledge them by saying them out loud. A win can be an affirmation.

Celebrate yourself!

CHAPTER 39

GET INTIMATE
WITH YOURSELF

INTIMACY IS MORE ABOUT YOU GETTING COMFORTABLE WITH yourself and expressing who you are than it is about anyone else. When you expose your true self in the presence of another person, this is true intimacy. This takes courage and trust in oneself to pull off.

We tend to think intimacy is more about exposing ourselves to someone else. It is, and it's also about exposing yourself to yourself first. What parts of you are you hiding from yourself? What parts are you hiding from everyone else?

It took me a long time to learn this one. I never looked at intimacy this way when I was younger, probably because I really didn't understand it. I was always feeling the need to hide myself and not show anyone the real me at the risk I'd be found out for who I really was and people wouldn't like that or they'd think I was really weird. So I did my best to fit in.

Well now I'm proud to say, yes, some people might not like parts of me, and others may think I'm weird, but that's okay. I'll admit I am weird, but that's what makes me me. And who isn't a little weird? I think we all secretly have some weirdness in us. I call this creative thinking and imagination.

You might say some of my favorite comedians are weird, but I assure you, people are not thinking they're weird; they're thinking, *This guy is funny.*

What I like about what comedians bring to the table is a level of imagination that has not yet been expressed. The great ones have a knack for putting opposing or unlikely associated realities together to make a situation really funny.

They invite their audience to look into who they really are in a way that is risky. That, my friends, is intimacy. Showing other people parts of yourself not because you're trying to please or perform but because that's what you enjoy doing. What lights you up. What you'd like to expose about yourself. How you'd like to express yourself.

True intimacy allows you to be yourself unapologetically. It's a vulnerable position to be in around another person, but that's why you have to get comfortable getting intimate with yourself first.

It's magical when you can do this. I remember continuously trying to hide the things I thought people wouldn't like about me, only to find out that these qualities are the very things that people love about me.

What a relief as a recovering perfectionist and people-pleaser. Looking at intimacy this way allowed me to explore who I am and how I wanted to express that in any given moment. I didn't act the way I believed other people wanted me to but instead gave way to what came through. I got comfortable with who that is and even surprised myself at times.

By allowing other people to have their own experience of you, you naturally open yourself up to your own authenticity and release the burden of pleasing people. You instead are able to turn pleasing people into giving, which does not have any strings attached, whereas pleasing others is a form of manipulation.

Only when we can become intimate with ourselves can we learn to give from the heart. With appreciation, love, and pleasure.

ACTION STEPS

How can you get intimate with yourself?

What are you hiding in order to fit in? Can you take off that mask for a day or a week to see how it feels? Can you have your own back when it feels scary? Can you practice allowing it to feel vulnerable until it feels good?

What sort of activities make you feel most like yourself? Can you do more of those so that joy enters your life? So that you feel joy with yourself? Get close to yourself, stay with it. It's a practice. Affirmations may be helpful here as we are becoming intimate with ourselves. "I am safe to be myself. I love myself."

CHAPTER 40

SHARE INSTEAD OF COMPARE

COMPETING AND COMPARING ARE PROBABLY SOME OF THE MOST common things we suffer from in our modern-day culture. With social media on the rise to becoming one of the only ways that younger people know how to connect, there also comes a severe disconnect.

Although it may start out as something playful, it eventually becomes a form of suffering for so many of us. The reason being that we rarely get the full story when we're looking at the end result of someone's success or only seeing the side of them they want to present to the world. There's no context for the journey this person has been on. This becomes problematic if we cannot hold space in ourselves for awareness around our own process and journey.

The truth is, none of us automatically find success without investing in ourselves first. What I mean by that is putting in the consistent focus, clarity, time, presence, energy, and love into what you truly want to create. This is what has to happen for anyone to become successful, no matter if it is creating a beautiful, healthy body or a thriving business.

The beauty of it is that it's also different for everyone. You can have someone teach you how they did it, but at the end of the day, it comes down to honoring your process. For myself, I call it the Allison way. It's my unique way of going about work, relationships, and life. If you want to forge a new path for yourself, you have to acknowledge that, yes, other people have really great ideas and strategies, but you also have a unique spin on how you'd like to implement it.

ACTION STEPS

Action Step 1

It's even valuable to define what success looks and feels like to you instead of taking on other peoples' definitions of success as your own. This is why it's so important to get clear on your desires and unapologetically ask for what you want because not everyone will find success the same way.

When we can do this, there's no competition and comparison because we begin to see our experience for the uniqueness that it has.

You sabotage yourself when your level of self-worth reflects what you see in other people. It's really hard to compete and compare when you have a high level of self-worth and appreciation for your own unique experience.

When you feel good about yourself, you generally want others to feel good too. You see others' successes as your past, present, or future successes, and you know how it feels to make your own desires a priority. You are sharing the feeling of success and lighting other people up, and they are lighting you up.

You see the power in lighting each other up or being inspired instead of needing what that person has or not feeling worthy. You no longer get pulled into the circle of dependence on a spiritual guru or coach for your happiness; you instead learn how to take inspired action. A good coach and spiritual teacher will teach you this.

Teach a person to fish. This is way more powerful.

When you're able to fill your needs in the self-worth department, life gets interesting. In my experience, there's less suffering, and there's a feeling of excitement. That's not to say issues of self-worth won't ever come up for you again, but the energy of them does dissipate. If you begin to pay attention to it and reflect on what could be going on deeper, then you gain valuable tools to navigate it.

For example, a very common thing we do is to get on social media and compare ourselves to other people. Whether they are super fit or successful in business, sometimes we get triggered when we see it. If this happens to you, ask yourself why. Is it about a need you are not meeting for yourself?

In my case, I was holding back in my career, making myself small, and then I'd get triggered when I'd see other fitness professionals doing what I secretly wished I could do. Only I wasn't doing those things or putting myself out there. It wasn't until I read the book *Daring Greatly* by Brené Brown that I realized if I wanted to stop comparing and blaming people, I needed to get into the arena myself.

So that's what I did. I started a podcast, I took an acting and improv class, I hired a business/energy coach, I worked on my voice, I took a creative writing class, I wrote this book, and the list goes on. I got into the arena of life and stopped making myself small. I started to take steps that were doable to become what I wanted to become.

You can do this too!

Action Step 2

What's the first step you can take to level up your self-worth? How do you want to express yourself? What does success feel like to you and your unique life? Write this down.

CHAPTER 41

INTEGRATE YOURSELF

You do not have to train like an athlete to think like one.

Holding space for our vision for ourselves and the potential we all have is a skill that is to be developed over time.

Every athlete knows this because they've learned to work consistently every day toward a bigger goal. They work little by little each week to make the bigger goal a reality. They can see the big picture when it comes to their body and the potential within mainly because they are living it.

It's not necessarily a superpower; it's that they've spent quality time testing the waters consistently. Because of this, they develop a sense of knowing what to expect long term. This is called persistence. It's the ability to keep going and having faith even if you cannot foresee the future. There is an inner knowing and confidence about what will happen.

Athletes know how to play the long game when it comes to their bodies. They've seen just about everything and have come across just about every injury, witnessing their body's recovery process. They learn on a deeper level how to support their body for better performance.

You can approach your body this way too. Approach your body's potential as something you're excited to learn more about and test the waters, so to speak. Start making yourself a priority and learn how to honor your body's process while pushing it to its limits—with awareness.

You may understand something but ask yourself if you have ever truly integrated it. Have you practiced it, tried it, felt it, implemented it, and lived it enough to really know it?

My client Suzanne learned this very lesson. When I first met Suzanne, she came to me thinking she should know how to do this already. She was putting unrealistic expectations on herself to know skills she hadn't yet trained for. She hadn't integrated the information; therefore, she wasn't able to know her true potential.

After experiencing some back issues, Suzanne came to me needing to come up with a plan of action for stabilizing and strengthening her back so that she'd not have these debilitating back spasms anymore. She wasn't having any luck with other trainers, so she came to me.

I taught her how to listen to what her body was telling her by going through key stretches and exercises and by paying attention to her body's signals. She started to realize that the smaller things that we implement on a daily basis add up to what actually supports us.

Soon after, she began to feel more confident and believed she could use these tools to get out of back pain if she needed to. She had more energy and was excited to come to the gym weekly for our sessions together. Suzanne's strength level increased, and she no longer experienced back pain when she'd take her walks and have to go up a steep hill. She was able to connect with the nuance of what fitness means to her, not to the average gym rat.

In her early sixties, she was able to redefine what fitness meant for her. Because she did this, she was able to take the judgment and the criticism out of the mix and truly own her experience of it.

ACTION STEP

Start creating a regular practice and test this out. Train yourself to begin integrating the information you take in or learn about yourself one step at a time. Take in only the information you need and start building a movement practice that brings greater awareness and satisfaction to yourself.

Be with it, feel it, and cherish it. This is how we move toward a greater goal and find joy in the process, not just the end result.

CHAPTER 42

IF YOU WANT TO CHANGE THE WORLD, START WITH YOURSELF

"YOU CAN'T SAVE OTHER PEOPLE FROM THEMSELVES," A COACH once told me. These words made perfect sense, and up until then, they had never occurred to me.

At that time, I'd been trying to save other people from themselves. My life felt hard because I was taking responsibility away from others and putting it unnecessarily on myself. What an impossible task.

Even though I look back on it and realize how exhausting it was at that time, I couldn't figure out why I was chronically fatigued and quite frankly not having much fun. I was taking myself way too seriously.

When I found the holy grail of wellness at the Chek Institute, I wanted to share what I'd learned with the world—only my approach was flawed. I wasn't giving people the opportunity to show up for themselves and own it. I was telling them that I had all the answers and to just listen to me because I knew what was best for them.

Well, if you can imagine, this didn't go over so well, and as a result, coaching people felt like a drag because I could never get people to do what I was asking them to do. I started to feel resistance in other people and then resentment in my job after a while. What started out being fun stopped being fun when I decided I'd save everyone.

What I hadn't realized at the time was that I needed to save myself, not everyone else. I needed to address my own shadows first before I could help anyone else.

I look back on it now with the words "righteous indignation." I'd just learned about all of these injustices that were going on behind the scenes in the food industry and the medical world, and I wanted to tell everyone about it. Surely sharing this information would get people on board with me without question, but I couldn't be more wrong about that.

As a coach, you learn that there's an art to guiding people to their own conclusions and hope for the best for them. You cannot save them from themselves; that's their job. You can only provide them with tools and guidance and trust that they will succeed. They ultimately have to forge their own path.

If you're a coach or a mentor to someone, ask yourself: Are you being honest with yourself? Are you humble? Are you curious?

It's less about knowing all the answers and more about you showing up for your client.

Most likely there's no one telling you that you have to know everything either. In my case, it was a story I made up about myself about what people expected of me. I made up an impossible scenario.

Lack of joy and fun is a sign that we are going about things in a heavy, unnecessary way. But people have been taught to work hard and to suffer, so it takes a while to unlearn that.

When I began handing responsibility over to the people I cared about when it came to their lives, I learned how to trust other people to take good care of themselves and to know what's right for them. I realized I could still guide a person and teach them how to guide themselves.

What a relief that was, knowing I could now focus on taking responsibility for my own life and knowing what's right for me. Everyone's happy—or better yet, everyone's responsible and accountable.

If you are a coach, this is the best advice I can give you. If you're not, you can still use this approach with your relationships.

ACTION STEP

Reflect on where in your relationships you may be taking responsibility away from others and putting it unnecessarily on yourself.

CHAPTER 43

THE VIBRATION OF SIMPLICITY AND EASE

"Why would I think about missing a shot I haven't taken yet?"

—Michael Jordan

DO YOU EVER NOTICE IF SOMETHING SEEMS TOO EASY, YOUR mind goes right to thinking, "Well that must not be right," or "Shouldn't it be harder than that?" I know mine does.

I've noticed that kind of talk in myself.

Many times, I've seen something so perfect present itself right in front of me, only to look for something else until I come full circle back to what originally came to me.

There's nothing wrong with making an informed decision, but when you constantly second-guess your own intuition, you lose trust in your ability and your inner knowing.

I had to learn how to trust my intuition by making decisions and trusting that it was the right decision for me. The more I was able to do this, the more trust I felt within myself.

Maybe it was even more about allowing myself to let life be fun and easy instead of doing it the hard way. The hard way was how I'd been taught to approach life. In my mind, if it wasn't hard work, it wasn't worth spending my energy on.

What a ridiculous notion. Where did this come from? It occurred to me that if I can make life hard, it's just as possible to make life easy. So that's what I did. I figured making life hard wasn't really working for me anymore, so why not try something different. I had nothing to lose. Remember when I mentioned I did things the Allison way? This is what I mean.

The crazy thing is that just acknowledging this and changing my belief about life created a whole new pattern of receiving for me. This reflected in my body, how I felt, and in things that were coming to me in my life.

I also realized that it was less about doing and pushing and more about allowing and supporting. Acknowledging how I truly wanted to live.

Simplicity and ease are a higher vibration. Complexity is a lower vibration.

Another aspect of this is waiting for the other shoe to drop. As I mentioned, one of the most influential books in my life has been *Daring Greatly* by Brené Brown. In this book, she explains the concept of foreboding joy, a "dress rehearsal for tragedy," and says that it is one of the most self-sabotaging behaviors we experience. It prevents us from being in the moment and experiencing true happiness. Foreboding joy prevents us from feeling anything at all and serves as a false sense of control.

Therefore, we focus on what could always go wrong. When we do this, we can never be in our heart space, only our heads. This creates tons of anxiety.

As Michael Jordan says, "Why would I worry about missing a shot I haven't taken yet?" Why worry about something that hasn't happened? Why not focus on what could go right instead of what could go wrong?

There's no risk to thinking this way, and trust me, life gets a whole lot easier if you do this. It's all just changing what you're focusing on—focusing on what you'd like to happen.

I'm not saying to stop paying attention to potential dangers or not use caution when needed. I'm saying decide what you'd like to focus on more often because focusing more on what could go wrong will never bring you happiness. It'll most likely bring you more things that could go wrong.

There is the notion of whether you are worthy of receiving the good in life, and that definitely plays a factor. There's also the reality of what we learned. Most of us learn how to forebode joy, thinking it's the more noble thing to do or that we'll somehow be able to control the situation better if we nip it in the bud.

The reality of this is that it is not going to help anyone, including yourself. With that, I invite you to begin thinking about how you can start focusing on what you'd like to happen in your life rather than what you'd not like to happen. The only reality there is the reality you are creating. Why not create the best work of art you can whip up?

Play with this, test it out, and see where it takes you. I came to the conclusion that this way of thinking was not serving me anymore. I'd run into the same issues over and over again, and after a while, I got so tired of it.

I remember having a conversation with myself in the car and thinking, *Well, what have we got to lose? We know this way's not working, might as well try something different. What's the risk? Maybe joy and bliss? Let's give it a try.*

So I did. I started listening to Abraham-Hicks recordings each day to get my mind in a more positive place. You see, you have to train your brain just like you have to train your body if you want to create a new pattern of thinking.

I found this to be incredibly enjoyable, and soon, I was doing the meditations daily, and then it became my routine. I started seeing synchronicities in my life, and I began realizing that it was only my perception that was holding me back.

Very soon after, I was contacted out of the blue by an incredible coach and mentor who I still work with to this day. She asked me if I'd like to work with her. At first, my ego said, "I don't need her help. I can do this on my own," but part of me realized that I did need her help because, as I mentioned earlier, you can't expect yourself to do things you haven't trained for or experienced yet. Little did I know there was so much I still needed to learn. It was a bit of a stretch for me at the time financially, but I took a leap of faith and started working with her.

This was one of my biggest first steps to learning how to receive. It was so uncomfortable for me to accept help because I'd been under the impression that I could do it all myself, not realizing that asking for help is one of the most powerful steps you can take in learning how to receive the good in life. It was also the first time I was able to take responsibility in a way that held me accountable on an energetic level. I had no idea this was possible or even something I could learn until I met Hanna.

She taught me how to manage my energy practically by increasing my sense of self-worth and expanding my energy out, making it bigger than any situation I was intimidated by. Using what's called family constellation therapy, she was able to guide me to heal my relationship with my parents, which ultimately helped me regain my trust in the universe to provide everything I needed and feel taken care of.

This was truly liberating for my soul. It's what led to the feeling of true safety and security, thus unlocking liberation for play and creative expression.

Call it the Universe, call it God, call it your higher self; it's really all the same. What's important is your perception of trust and the feeling of being taken care of. When we can lean into this and clear what's blocking us from feeling this, which is natural, we can begin to realize our true potential and begin to trust ourselves. We can feel worthy and whole again, knowing we can relax because everything we need is in our perception. Now that's true health.

How can you begin to retrain your brain to see the goodness in life?

Energy statements are a great way to open yourself up to possibilities. They're different from affirmations as they allow you to become open to all possibilities of how life could unfold for you. All of us have expectations of how our dreams will come to fruition. Energy statements are a great tool for setting the tone for your energy and an opportunity for you to let go of how your scenario will play out.

Change your frequency to match what you'd like to happen. Then you can begin to connect to the feeling of your situation as if it's already happened and get excited about the potential of how it'll happen. In a way, you let yourself off the hook and allow yourself to receive and the Universe to provide.

Examples:

What would it take for me to...

- Be in a body I feel great in?

- Have an abundant amount of energy every day?

- Love the body I'm living in?

- Feel grounded and connected every day?

- Feel like I'm taken care of?

- Trust that I'll be taken care of?

- Have delicious, high-quality food?

- Enjoy my life to its fullest?

ACTION STEPS

Write down three to five energy statements. You can use my examples or come up with one more specifically suited for yourself. Repeat them to yourself out loud as often as you can. I will usually repeat them three to five times every morning. You can repeat them as much as you'd like. This will set a new tone for what you want to create without you having to stress out about how it will happen.

CHAPTER 44

HOW DO YOU DIGEST YOUR LIFE?

HOW IS YOUR BODY RESPONDING TO YOUR LIFE? HOW DOES YOUR body respond to your environment, life changes, your beliefs, the beliefs of others around you, etc.? Are you enjoying life, seeing the goodness all around you, taking the time to acknowledge your small wins or the beautiful subtleties?

Think about where you are holding resistance and tension in your body. Could this be an indication that you're slowing your ability to receive and assimilate the goodness in life for fear that you might actually get what you want or because of a belief you have about yourself or the world? Is it a need to feel supported or nurtured in your life?

We hold tension without realizing the deeper aspect of it. Then one day, we end up with a digestive issue and wonder if it's something we're eating. We rarely look at our lifestyle and our beliefs about ourselves.

The question is, are you paying attention?

I once had a good friend tell me how well you digest your food is a reflection of how well you digest your life. It makes sense if you think about how our emotions affect our physical bodies.

The point my friend was making is that many times, our digestive system reflects what we could be feeling about our life. How we either receive or reject our life.

Believe me, I've been there many times. Parts of me are afraid of change. Not because it's bad; it's that oftentimes, it's a bit unknown what the change might actually be. I feel like most of us are in this same boat. We haven't really learned to navigate the unknown in life.

The good news is that you can identify how you're digesting life from your actual digestive system; this allows you to make changes in your life. For example, coming up with a plan for play and creativity. I once coached one of my clients to have impromptu dance parties either by herself or with her kids as part of her home play.

She was in a holding pattern of doing it right all of the time, aka perfectionism, and this was holding her back. It was slowing her digestive system, her metabolic rate, and her thyroid.

I explained to her that you have to start learning how to play again. Give yourself permission to make a mistake and make light of it. Dance like no one's watching and play with your oracle cards as much as you'd like.

This energy allows us to relax within the structure we've set up for ourselves. It goes back to the two energies I talked about in the beginning of this book, the masculine and the feminine. She had to learn how to harness her healthy feminine along with her healthy masculine.

This reflects in your body as flexibility, relaxation, and enjoying the good in life. Only then can you fully be in rest and digest mode, otherwise known as your body's parasympathetic nervous system.

ACTION STEPS

You can even go so far as to change your meal environment up by eating by candlelight, sitting on the floor, or making a habit to eat as a family every night or eat with no distractions. Try eating with your fork in the other hand for a change, or eat with chopsticks. This'll get you out of your thinking mode and put you in a more creative, relaxed state. It will literally change your neural pathways, making you more innovative in the long run.

CHAPTER 45

REKINDLE YOUR INNER CREATIVITY

I REALLY THINK THAT WHAT WE'VE BEEN MISSING IS PLAY. ONE of my favorite books, *The Artist's Way* by Julia Cameron, led me to where I am now. When I read it, I lit up like a supernova. My artist woke up like a sleeping giant ready to go. I felt like this book had been written for me, confirming my own story of the repressed artist.

How many of us are repressing our artists out of the need to belong, fit in, and perform? I was definitely doing this. I'd been doing this most of my life and was still doing this.

I couldn't believe that at the age of forty-seven, I could still live out my dream as an artist. Here I was thinking these are things I needed to develop when I was younger, thinking it's too late to do it now. I thought everything that came out needed to be perfect right out of the gate. Boy, was I wrong.

I didn't realize the work is just getting it all out and then looking at what you have. Here I was, thinking it had to be in this perfect little package, all ready to go. Writing for me soon became a pleasure, something I looked forward to every morning.

I realized that if everything needed to be perfect right out of the gate, there'd be no nuanced experience of my creation process. We'd never learn anything about ourselves.

Honestly, my experience of writing a book has probably been my greatest act of self-development in my entire life so far. It kind of feels like the pinnacle of self-development. Many of my thoughts, insights, and stories are out on paper, and I get to process these as I go.

The truth is, it's never too late to discover your inner creativity. Also, what is this idea of perfection we are weighing ourselves down with? Remember the woman who was in her nineties still working on herself? Improving her emotional resilience, continuing to connect with herself?

My friends, I'm here to tell you that it never ends. It's infinite.

A fire had been lit in me, and as a result, I started writing for fifteen minutes every morning. This then turned into thirty minutes and then one hour every morning. I wrote about whatever was coming to mind without judgment and without censoring myself. This is how I wrote this book.

I wouldn't have believed it myself if you'd told me a year ago, but it happened, and it happened fast. When we're able to stop editing ourselves and start expressing ourselves through play, the sky's the limit as to what we can do with that. Our experience becomes easier, lighter, and more fun as well.

ACTION STEPS

How can you reconnect with your creativity? What did you love to do as a child?

What activity have you wanted to try but were afraid you may not be great at right off the bat? What feels expansive and playful? Painting, writing, dancing, collaging, beautifying your space, singing, learning an instrument? Our creativity is our magic. You can tap into this at any time.

CHAPTER 46

GETTING HEALTHY IS LIKE LEARNING HOW TO RIDE A BIKE

HEALTH IS A JOURNEY; HOWEVER, ONCE YOU DISCOVER WHAT works for you, you'll never forget how to do it. It takes as long as it takes, but if you're willing to explore and get curious about what could work for your body and explore the spiritual aspects of health, you'll discover a connection with yourself that is unshakable.

This is because you've done the work of building a foundation. Your foundation is your framework that never waivers and that also allows you to change certain patterns with the seasons.

Things like blood sugar regulation and the right amount of movement and food intake become something you know about yourself instead of being a mystery.

That way, if you experience chaos outside of you, you'll have a calm disposition inside. You'll be better prepared to handle the stresses of life with resilience.

Consistency is key.

You are your practice.

Learning what your body needs and then paying attention to that is your practice.

Nicole couldn't figure out why it was so hard to get healthy. She was running into so many blocks when it came to food. Nicole had also been struggling with an eating disorder for some time now. Associating complexity with getting healthy, she just assumed that she needed to do a laundry list of tasks to get to where she wanted to be and feel better.

What she didn't realize was that it was all about her bringing to light what was actually happening. You see, anxiety happens for most of us when we try to solve a problem by shooting in the dark.

This is a surefire way of never knowing what works and what doesn't. Yet we waste so much valuable energy on trying to do so much when we could first just take a look at what we're doing and see how we can tweak it to better support us.

Looking at her food log, I told her that she was not eating enough to be able to provide herself with the energy she needed to sustain her life. This could be why she was feeling overwhelmed and anxious most of the time. I suggested she start eating breakfast every morning, and then we built on that. She was taken aback by this and yet was perplexed by how simple this solution was.

Even though part of her felt like surely there was more to this, she followed through with eating breakfast every morning. It was a challenge for her because she'd been skipping breakfast for so long that her body needed time to adjust by curbing her high adrenaline levels in the morning with food. Starting the day with a light and easily digestible breakfast was exactly what Nicole needed. She immediately began feeling like she had more energy and motivation. Her disposition in life was more optimistic, and she was better able to handle and move forward with healing much of her personal trauma.

She was even able to heal her relationship with dance. Dance was something that started out as a joy for her when she was young but became painful later as she experienced the pitfalls of perfectionism.

Because she was able to heal her relationship with food and make it fun, simple, and joyful again, she healed her relationship with both her body and her movement. What was incredible for me to witness was that after all this, Nicole created a business that helps other people heal their relationship with their body with dance. She was able to reconnect with her movement signature and expression, and now she's teaching others how to do that too.

How incredible is that!

It was all because she decided she'd be open to learning a new skill and assessing what she was doing without judgment or criticism.

Nicole's willingness to look at what was not working and then take inspired action to implement what could work allowed her to finally find peace in knowing what she was doing was supporting her needs. She was able to reap the benefits of consistently feeling more grounded, calm, and connected in her body. Nicole learned what truly works for her. This is what joy looks like.

ACTION STEPS

How can you support yourself?

- Suggestions: Eat breakfast, eat smaller meals more frequently, embrace simplicity.

- List one to three behavior patterns related to your health that you'd like to release.

- List one to three behavior patterns related to your health that work for you.

CHAPTER 47

RECLAIMING YOUR PERSONAL POWER

WHERE DOES YOUR PERSONAL POWER RESIDE?

The secret to reclaiming your power is in your acknowledgment of parts of yourself both physical and energetic, your level of compassion for yourself, and your ability to allow what needs to come through.

You can start by literally feeling in your body where your personal power resides. Also ask yourself, *Where am I suppressing my personal power?* This is a matter of where you might feel pain or tension in your body. That may be a really big clue as to where you are holding or resisting.

It's okay if you've been doing this for some time. Many times, we develop tension in our bodies from trauma we experienced when we were young. For me, this was the case. My story is a rite-of-passage, coming-of-age scenario.

I discovered I was suppressing my personal power right between my eyes, otherwise known as your Ajna Chakra or third eye. This was so interesting to me because it's where intuition lives.

As a young woman around the age of twelve, I stopped trusting my intuition. As a result, I developed allergies and sinus issues at that age.

My parents sent me to an ear, nose, and throat specialist, and I received allergy shots every week to a few times a month. I kept this going until I was in my twenties. When I had kids, I all of a sudden didn't need the monthly shots anymore and haven't needed them since.

When I look back on it, of course I numbed out that part of my body to survive. I learned at a young age that if I was going to belong to my family and be accepted by their friends, I could no longer be frank and honest about what I was seeing in other people. It would come off as rude, and my parents would be somewhat embarrassed by me voicing my insights about other people's actions.

I was just sharing what came to mind. I thought I was being helpful. But other people did not experience me this way, and over time, I didn't feel like anyone was listening to me, so I became extremely frustrated and angry. If I wanted to fit in, I figured I better get with the program, and I stopped listening to that part of me.

The cost was tremendous both physically and energetically. When I hit my twenties, it was a shit show. I felt like I was having a crisis of self, which was also a result of retiring from gymnastics and graduating from college. I'd lost the identity I'd had for most of my youth. I was no longer a student or an athlete.

With nothing to fill the void, I was left feeling like the rug had been pulled out from under me, feeling instantly depressed and unworthy.

I felt that I'd done everything I was supposed to do, but I still didn't feel whole; there was still something missing,

I left my self-esteem back at age twelve and never looked back. I sacrificed a valuable part of myself to fit in, and let me tell you, it was exhausting.

Where do you feel your power in your body? Are you able to release the tension in some areas by acknowledging them, thanking them, and then inviting them back into the whole?

Only then can we connect with our personal power. Physical symptoms don't just show up out of thin air. Most likely they've been there for a while. It's your body's way of communicating with you and getting your attention. Some of us pay attention, and others do not.

I believe that many of these things are deeper and come from a place of dissociation from ourselves out of the perceived need to belong and feel loved. Once you can become aware of your own unique power and where that comes from, you can finally move toward a sense of wholeness and lasting wellness. A feeling of trust, clarity, and focus. Feeling strong, powerful, and light.

257

What does power represent to you? Can you think of anything that symbolizes that for you?

Is it a strong, stable body or a color? Is it feeling beautiful? Is it feeling acknowledged?

The question is, what is that for you? This becomes a great journey to search that out and discover it for ourselves.

I've always felt if I can connect with my inner child, acknowledge her, and bring her back into the whole, I can do anything. My personal power comes from connecting with my play, creative expression, and curiosity. This all traces back to pure innocence.

ACTION STEP

Listen to the "Connecting with Your Body" meditation.

Go to www.finallythrivingbook.com to download this meditation.

CHAPTER 48

VIRTUES VS. RIGHTEOUS INDIGNATION

"The highest virtue is not virtue and therefore really is virtue. But inferior virtue cannot let go of being virtuous and therefore is not virtue."

—Lao Tzu

A VIRTUE IS A STRENGTH. IT'S SOMETHING THAT IS NOT CONSCIOUS of itself.

What a concept in this day and time of virtue signaling. To be virtuous is literally to not know you are virtuous.

In his talk, "The Road to Hell Is Paved with Good Intentions," Alan Watts translated this quote into, "The highest virtue is not conscious of itself as virtue and therefore really is virtue."

It's like a butterfly. The butterfly's not aware of how beautiful it is or that it can fly, that it inspires beauty in everyone that witnesses it. Our body and its process of regeneration are virtues. Do you see the magnificence in that, or do you take it for granted?

On the other hand, righteous indignation is the need to make another person or group wrong and yourself or your group right. A reaction to a sense of personal injustice.

Alan Watts also said, "How do you know what's good for other people? How do you know what's good for you?"

I think virtues have been confused with righteous indignation. If a virtue is not aware of itself, then what the heck is virtue signaling about? Well, I think it's about our inherent need to make others wrong and ourself right. Our deep need to prove and defend. These are just unresolved issues within ourselves.

I invite you to think about it this way. What if, when you feel the need to make others wrong and yourself right, you are actually denying parts of yourself? You're not allowing yourself to be completely you because what if you change your mind and suddenly you agree with that person. Who are you then?

What if you decide to agree to disagree with that person? How liberating would that be for both people?

Realizing that everyone has their own unique experience of life and that you don't have to agree with everyone you come across, relating to each other with respect instead of the need to make another person wrong—now that's powerful.

This could take your relationships to a whole new level. One of understanding and compassion.

ACTION STEPS

Do you see the value in that? Practice this by saying, "Let's agree to disagree," to people you do not agree with. Can you still respect and honor that person's opinion even though you disagree with their perspective? Better yet, could this open the door for you to see more of where they are coming from? That can bring a whole new level of compassion into the mix.

Reflect on where you see any discrepancies within yourself when you disagree or are triggered by another person's perspective.

CHAPTER 49

BE YOUR OWN SUPERHERO

STEPPING INTO YOUR PERSONAL POWER CAN BE VERY MUCH LIKE reconnecting with your inner superhero. Not so much in the way of externally saving the world but more like saving yourself first. Like I said earlier, you can't save anyone from themselves, it's an illusion. You can only save yourself, so why not be your own superhero?

Acknowledging parts of myself, I've found, is my greatest superpower. What do I mean when I say parts of myself? I mean that we all have parts of ourselves that are conflicted, and that's normal. We see that externally when we come across people who trigger us. That essentially is a sign that there are parts of you that are conflicted.

Listening and learning how to love these parts has been the work. It takes observing yourself, not so much identifying with your emotions but allowing them to move through to see this. Acknowledge these conflicting parts of yourself and bring them back into the whole.

It's much like the work of an actor. The actor harnesses the energy of the character they are working with, and then after their work is done, they move on to another character. It's not that they forget about that character.

They have experienced the essence of that character with great reverence, and now that essence becomes a part of them. This part is not necessarily in the driver's seat, but it's a part of the whole that makes them up as a person.

This is how you work too; you just might not know it yet. I think that could be why we're so fascinated with actors: because we see our own process expressed by them and may even secretly wish we could express all parts of ourselves without judgment like they do.

The good news is that you can! When an emotion comes up, notice if you feel the need to suppress it or express it. If you're not ready to express it, that's okay; just notice that first. After a while, try expressing it and notice how that feels. For example, we don't really get permission to express our anger very often, but if you can express it in the moment, you can liberate yourself.

This is why we now have rage rooms. It's because we need to express these emotions in the moment so we don't build resentment. Otherwise, they just get stuck in our body and eventually come out with greater intensity.

Unexpressed emotions can also lead to disease. I've seen people living for other people so much so that they manifest chronic fatigue or fibromyalgia in their bodies. This is also a side effect of siphoning off too much of your energy.

Too much unexpressed anger can manifest as heart problems because we are holding on to too much resentment, heartbreak, and pain. Cancer manifests from unexpressed emotions that are eating away at you, and the list goes on.

If you're like me and learned at a very young age that it's safer to hide your emotions from everyone, then I have good news. You can learn how to feel and express these emotions again. It just takes practice. It may feel a little messy in the beginning, but the more you begin to get comfortable with who you are and how you express yourself, the better you'll feel.

When we can gain the ability to play with our emotions like performance art, it is magical. Like any performance artist, you let other people be responsible for their own responses or reactions to your expression. That's the magical part.

You never know how you will affect other people, but here's a secret: you could never control that anyway. So why not stop trying to control that and just be you? It's both scary and liberating to give yourself permission to be unapologetically you.

ACTION STEPS

What parts of yourself are conflicted? Can you bring awareness to them? Can you name them?

Once you notice those parts, instead of shaming them or turning away from them, can you love them? Can you be gentle with the tension? Can you let these parts move through your body with expression? How would this look for you?

CHAPTER 50

THE NEED TO BELONG IS STRONG

OUR NEED TO BELONG AND BE LOVED IS SO POWERFUL. EVERY one of us had a deep need to belong to our family when we were younger and still do. Most of us did things to fit in by changing our behavior because that need is so strong. In doing this, we compromised our true selves in the hopes of fitting in and belonging to our family. This is what we do in order to feel loved.

It's not all bad. Many of the things we did were so we could learn about life. But as I mentioned earlier, our values do break off and change as we get older, and some of the things we learned when we were young may no longer work for us.

This is because when we become adults, we are responsible for filling our own needs.

If we are feeling deeply that we're going against our family's values, this may create the deeper need to belong. Which can sometimes happen unexpectedly if you're changing your values or beliefs about desires in your life. This can come up as a block for some people if we are fearing subconsciously that we'll no longer belong to our family if we move forward with a desire that doesn't fit the family values.

This even comes up in our society. Groupthink is a deep-seated need to belong to the tribe. It's a survival mechanism, and it's very strong.

What do you desire?

What a question! How often do you get asked this question, and how often do you ask yourself this question? I struggled with this at first because I never really allowed myself to entertain this question, not realizing how this relates to everything I'm creating in my life.

I struggled with it because I was afraid to commit to something I might be disappointed about. I did this for so long that eventually I talked myself into a reality with a very controlled set of wants. I made my wants and myself small to fit my limited beliefs about myself.

I stopped using my imagination, and so then my potential piddled out and stayed limited within my controlled beliefs about what I wanted. I eventually got to a point where I suppressed my wants so much I didn't even know what I wanted anymore.

Now that's not to say I didn't find success, I did, but it was short-term success, not big-picture success. I was not playing the long game with my wants, not acknowledging my true desires. Meaning, I truly want to have goodness in my life not just some of the time but all of the time. The power of living with intention is key to that.

I've learned to practice how to allow myself to acknowledge and discern those wants, asking myself, are they mine or someone else's?

It's important, especially if you live with someone and you both share wants together. Much like values, you can share them, but it's super important to be discerning with your wants aside from your partner's because you're going to have those too.

It's also important to differentiate your short-term wants from your long-term desires. Desires to me are messages from the divine that move you toward your greater purpose in life. Short-term wants may be confused with other people's wants or their projections onto you. You mistake them for yours, or you may not know yourself well enough to know what your wants are, and so you grab onto someone else's or what you perceive as societal or family wants. This is where we go wrong and why people get what they want materially and then do not feel satisfied or still feel like something is missing.

The best way I've found to tune in to this is to begin daydreaming about what your life would look and feel like if you actually got what you wanted. When you get a feel for it, it becomes easier to navigate.

Once you start getting what you want, you'll begin to notice things you get that aren't really your wants, as opposed to the wants of

others, from the feeling you get from the outcome. You can then
begin to decide if what you want is truly what you want.

If when you get what you want, it fills a deep desire within you
and creates abundant energy and creativity, then you know
you're on to something. If, however, you get what you want and
you feel depressed or not fulfilled, then you may be missing the
mark. This is a good sign that you have only tapped into your
surface-level basic needs and have not yet tuned into your true
desires. It's totally okay if this is you; rarely does anyone teach us
how to discern between the two.

The mind wants to keep us safe, and so it will try to talk us out
of things. This is why it is so important to *feel* into our wants.
The heart knows. The soul knows. The body knows. The brain is
tricky; it needs to be trained.

What this could be telling you is that there may be some more
work to be done there. Pay most attention to what your inner
child is telling you. All your unmet needs when you were young
must be met by you as an adult now for you to fully realize your
ultimate desire potential.

Needy adults only get what they want and need more. If there
is an insatiable need to want more, then that tells you to pay
attention to what your inner child is trying to communicate to
you. It may be more about getting an emotional need met by
just giving yourself some attention and acknowledging your
emotions.

ACTION STEPS

What do you want? What do you really want? Sit with this question. Walk with it. Run with it. Feel into the question, and don't be afraid of the answer.

Make a list of what you desire for yourself and your life. Not what your family wants, your peers want, your community wants, but what you want. Just you. Include what this feels and looks like. Make sure to include every detail about the experience you are having when your desires come to fruition.

CHAPTER 51

INTEGRATE YOUR RECEIVING AND GIVING BODY

YOUR BODY HAS A FEMININE, OR RECEIVING, SIDE AND A masculine, or giving, side.

Do you ever notice how the right and left sides of your body interact with each other?

Do you have more injuries on the right or left side of your body? Where are you focusing most of your attention from doing or being? Are you a good receiver? How do you receive love? Do you listen? How do you express love? Do you support yourself and others? How do you rest?

It's crucial to become aware of how you're giving and receiving life. At some point, this needs to be a balance for you. So many of my clients have come to me wanting to do more when, really, they need less.

Health becomes this complex puzzle they are constantly needing to fix or solve. This is so hard to be with and, after a while, just not much fun. Looking at our bodies from the perspective of duality and how these two energies can work together, in my opinion, is way more fun. Sure, we need to know how our body works practically and how to support it, but we also must learn to let go of the constant struggle to know everything. There is balance.

This is where your feminine and masculine parts come in. Your left side of your body is your feminine or receiving side, and your right side is your masculine or giving side. Your left brain is connected to your masculine, logical side, and your right brain is connected to your feminine, creative side.

This is why when exercising, you must have some kind of cross pattern movements to integrate these two sides. A cross pattern movement is any move in which you are using your opposite arm and leg in unison, which is very helpful at integrating your right and left brain.

Just think about how most people go about their day. Most are sitting in one position, for the most part, in front of a screen. There's not much movement integration and so not much brain integration.

Yes, the good news is that some movements can integrate your brain and bring these two parts together. If you feel like doing these exercises is like chewing gum and patting your belly while balancing a spinning plate on a stick, then you probably really need them in your life.

Movement is an excellent way to integrate your right and left brain and put you back in a creative mode again. Another kind of movement practice that brings your body together is what I call sequencing. I also teach my clients how to do this as it builds resilience in the nervous system, much like playing music, if you've ever played an instrument.

You start out with simple movements and then continue to make the movements a little more complex each time you go up and down the floor with them. This kind of work will make you stronger, create more balance, turn on all of your stability muscles, and my favorite part, help your brain work better.

This is also an excellent way to build your nervous system up without depleting your body and energy reserves. As a trainer, I've learned about many different ways of going about a workout depending on the person I've been working with.

If someone needs to build resilience in their nervous system, I'll have them integrate their brain with some key cross patterning exercises to start and then move on to sequencing their movement. This will allow them to first get their mind out of the mix and then build on what they can respond to by slowly adding on more.

It's very much like when I'd take drumming class, and I'd start with a sequence of beats. Another person would come in with a different sequence while I continued on, and then we'd continue to add more instruments into the mix until we'd all be playing in unison, and we'd continue until we couldn't anymore.

You can do this with your movement too. It's exhausting, but in a different way than you'd be exhausted from, say, your standard strength training workout. It's more energizing, and you walk away with more resilience and dexterity. Your brain can now integrate more movement, which in the long run is less stressful on the body.

ACTION STEPS

Try a cross pattern move daily to integrate your right and left brain. Here's one you can try:

Start on your hands and knees with your back in a neutral position. Inhale and extend your opposite arm and leg out away from your body. Then exhale and bring your opposite arm and knee toward each other while letting your back round a little. Repeat this slowly for five to ten repetitions on each side.

Simple Exercise Sequence

1. Start by balancing on one foot and pulling your knee toward your chest. Keeping your chest upright, extend your standing leg and hip fully and ground your foot. Hold this for a few seconds or until you feel balanced and then alternate to the next side. Alternate each side five times.

2. Grab your foot with your hand on that same side behind you so that you are stretching the front of your leg while

balancing on the other side and reaching up with your other hand. Squeeze your buttocks and open the hip while aligning the knees and tucking the hips under. Make sure you are activating your abdominals too. Hold for a few seconds or until you feel balanced and then switch to the other side. Alternate each side five times.

3. Rotate your feet and toes toward each other while standing, and with a slight bend in the knees, reach down toward your toes. Repeat with your toes facing away from each other. Alternate each side five times.

4. Bring your feet wide apart from each other and shift your weight from one side to the other with a lunge to one side. Bend one knee as you shift and extend the other. Do this slow and gradually; do not overextend your inner thigh line. Extend just enough that feels right for you. Feel a gentle stretch in your inner thigh line.

Do this sequence at the beginning of each workout to activate and stretch your body.

Go to www.finallythrivingbook.com for these movement videos.

CHAPTER 52

YOU ARE UNLIMITED POTENTIAL

MOST OF US ONLY PERCEIVE WHAT WE KNOW, EXPERIENCE, OR have been told. Rarely do we think outside the box to what could be possible, especially when it comes to the potential of our body. In health and wellness, we're left with limited possibilities most of the time. We attach to old stories about our bodies and take way too much consideration of other so-called experts in health.

This severely limits possibility. When it comes to healing, getting stronger, and performing better, your imagination will get you there. You have to be open to the possibility that you can make it. That's why practice and showing up for yourself are so important because they demonstrate your desired potential.

No one knows your potential; only you do. That's why it's important to work with people who believe in you and will support you in a way that will lift you up rather than bringing you down or telling you what you can't do.

I'm not saying we don't have limitations. We certainly do, but there is possibility beyond the limitations we perceive in the physical.

I've pretty much seen it all. One client of mine came in with both hips and knees replaced and having had surgery from cancer in her abdominal area. She had been through so much in that year, but she was determined to get strong. Within her physical limits, she was able to dispel her fear of reinjury and create stability again in her legs and hips.

Her accomplishments were that she was now able to feel her hamstrings and glutes as she walked up the stairs, whereas before, she always felt like she was going to fall backward. She gradually got herself out of much of the pain she was experiencing too.

She was able to feel her abs working despite the big scar and numbness she had experienced prior. She did this by showing up for herself every week and following through with her practice. By honoring her body.

She never thought this was possible until she found the right person to guide her and started doing the work. That's the beauty of it. We rarely look at these experiences as exploring our unlimited potential, but that's what they are.

What if she had had a doctor to tell her, "You'll never be able to heal or get stronger, so you might as well give up now," or "Why bother? You'll just go downhill from here without any improvement." It happens all the time, and people believe it, whether it's a doctor, friend, or family member.

We tend to believe it when someone tells us a condition has been passed down to us or when someone tells us about their perceived limitations we have. My question is, how could they possibly know? The answer is there's no way they can. They can only give you their opinion. This includes doctors.

The problem is that we take this information to heart as our truth. Get this: we are so powerful we literally manifest what people tell us we are. How crazy is that?

Why not test the waters and start cultivating the beliefs about yourself you'd like to have?

Now please don't think that I'm saying not to follow your doctor's advice; please do what feels right for you. But how many times have doctors been wrong? They are human like anyone else, they make mistakes, and they are in the "practice" of medicine.

You can begin to treat doctors as consultants for your body. Take their advice with a grain of salt, so to speak, because you are ultimately your own authority over your body. No one else. Find a doctor who shares your values.

This will make a huge difference in your health because you'll have someone in your corner who will support you in your health journey. That's ultimately what we all want: support.

ACTION STEP

How do you want to be supported in your health? What do you need?

Write down the qualities of the people you desire as your health consultants.

This can include medical doctors, alternative health doctors, physical therapists, coaches, and personal trainers.

CHAPTER 53

WALKING THE LABYRINTH

One of the biggest obstacles we place upon ourselves when learning something new is the perspective that learning is linear. Has anyone taught you an alternative? For most of us, no.

I couldn't figure out why my clients would get so bummed about not being able to master something they just learned within that week or month. They were left criticizing themselves for not getting to the next perceived level with it. Or saying, "I should know how to do this," when they've never done it before or despite the fact that they have yet to explore all aspects that lesson had to offer.

Of course, we feel like we should know how to do this already. After all, we're living in our bodies. There's a level of bewilderment around why we don't know how to take care of our body, but navigating your body is a skill to develop just like anything else. Especially if you weren't taught how to do this when you were growing up.

I remember feeling frustrated as a coach not knowing how to convey the importance of experiencing all aspects of health to my clients and what that feels like for each person.

Early on in my career, I got bored with the basics of fitness and health, and so I searched to find more. I realized my clients needed to know the basics, and they also needed to know what was beyond that, so I brought them a more nuanced version of health and wellness. My own health journey was truly magical, and I wanted all my clients to experience this for themselves.

Then one day, it occurred to me that learning is not linear—it's circular. It's actually spiraling and oscillating back and forth. Much like your Chakras, or your energy centers.

What we forget is that we're all on a journey of discovering our true selves. When we forget this, we tend to feel stuck, and our life feels static. Only life is not static; it's dynamic, and for most people, we feel generally safer when we stick with what we know.

At some point, sticking to what we know stops working, and we get that feeling of wanting to grow and expand, only it doesn't always feel safe. That's when you have that "come to Jesus" moment and realize what you're doing is not working anymore, and the need to change and grow becomes greater than your need to stick with what you know.

This is where I come into my client's life. They're feeling stuck, and they're not sure what to do. They know intuitively that something has to change, but they're not sure how to go about it. They feel stuck, unhappy, and oftentimes in physical pain. They seek a new way of looking at their health journey and wish to connect with their body on a deeper level. A way that creates lasting awareness and change.

The labyrinth has been a symbol for my business for some time now as it represents for me the way I approach my teachings and how I coach my clients. During the learning process, it can be perceived that we go back to square one at times or have to start back at the beginning. That's never the case. You'll never go back to square one; you're just spiraling down to pick up other aspects of the same experience so you can perceive it differently. This is magical.

Traditionally, the labyrinth symbolizes a person's rite of passage or initiation, if you will. According to the Veriditas, walking the labyrinth involves three phases: purgation, illumination, and union.

First comes the path of releasing what no longer serves you, creating a catalyst for change. Next, you're spending time in the center, where you begin learning how to receive the goodness in life. Finally, you return as your transformed self with a new perception, experiencing the world in a new way.

There are layers of perception to every experience. That's what makes life fun. You might learn something different the next time you're faced with that same situation, or a skill you've done a million times may have a different purpose the millionth time you do it.

Who knows what could come out of it, but where we go wrong is thinking of progress exponentially going up instead of expanding. You'll dip down at times, but it's to pick up new information or have a different experience of the same thing. Maybe it's something you'd like to master in your life. In his book, *Outliers*, Malcolm Gladwell says you must put in 10,000 hours of deliberate practice to actually master something.

That's why always going back to the basics in the way of movement and nutrition is crucial for experiencing the layers of learning within. You probably remember the movie *The Karate Kid* (if you're younger, maybe not) and the iconic scene where Mr. Miyagi has Daniel wash the windows and wax his car, giving him the mantra, "Wax on, wax off."

Daniel clearly perceived this as nonsensical, boring work. He dismissed its value in the moment and got frustrated and angry that Mr. Miyagi was neglecting to teach him what Daniel thought he was there for. Little did he know, he was training to take the mind out of it. Daniel was training his intuition, and over time, he didn't even have to think about the moves, his body just moved intuitively for him.

If you think about it, yoga is based on this same principle too. At the core of its essence, yoga is a practice of self-union. There are only so many moves that you can learn. You essentially do the same moves over and over again. How don't we get bored with that, then?

Because you're experiencing them differently each time. But you'd never know these depths of experiences until you repeated these same moves over and over again. You're essentially taking your monkey mind out of the equation. This is why yoga's original purpose was a practice to prepare a person for meditation.

It's a normal part of the process to feel like we're spiraling backward. The problem is that we've not been taught how to navigate this, much less that it even exists. That awareness just hasn't been developed yet.

Therefore, we're left with the feeling of not doing enough, not being enough, or feeling frustrated because we took a perceived step back. Only this is not what's happening at all.

The ego loves to move in a linear fashion and wants to know exactly what to expect next. When we can learn how to take the mind out of dominating the situation in our learning process, we can go so much further with less effort.

I see energy in motion. I watch people move literally every day. It's been my profession for almost twenty years now. Before that, I was a gymnast and then a gymnastics coach, so you could say I have an eye for movement.

I say this because when I picture my business and what it looks like energetically, I picture it as a labyrinth, spiraling down, allowing my clients to let go of what's no longer needed, taking in new information in the middle and then spiraling back out to integrate, practice, and share.

This is a process we all go through with everything we learn, and what I love about it is that there's no need to criticize yourself, nothing is lost, and there's always continuous expansion. It's a beautiful process, and it's one of the most natural processes we go through as humans in our creative journey.

ACTION STEP

How can you take the idea of walking the labyrinth and apply it to your learning process? How would that allow you to see yourself differently?

CHAPTER 54

THE CRUMBLING

"There are no ordinary moments."

—Dan Millman, *Peaceful Warrior*

When I was a gymnast, I remember so clearly thinking my ability to do gymnastics was what set me apart from everyone else. I thought it was what made me special. I remember thinking, *Wow, I can do things that not many people can do, and people are so impressed by that.* The feeling was incredible.

The problem with that way of thinking is that when you are not able to do those tricks anymore, the skills that set you apart from everyone else and made you special, who are you then, and what makes you special?

Peaceful Warrior is a story of a college-aged male gymnast who has an incredible life-changing experience. In the beginning, he has an insatiable sense of invincibility, as most of us do when we're young. He's a gymnast who's pushing the limits of the physical and winning.

Dan Millman, the main character in the movie, which is based on his book, *Way of the Peaceful Warrior*, ends up being somewhat reckless with his sense of invincibility and crashes his motorcycle, injuring himself severely. Lucky enough to survive, he picks up the pieces of himself and goes through all the stages of grief. He gets angry and disgruntled, and he quickly falls into depression, feeling sorry for himself and what he once was.

No longer is he capable physically of doing what he once could do. He has to settle into the idea that he won't be going back to that life anymore.

At the beginning of the story, Dan meets a mysterious man who claims he can teach him the way of the peaceful warrior and takes him on as his student. Dan calls him Socrates, and he appears to be real, although you never really know because Socrates will appear and then disappear as soon as Dan turns his head. This mysterious man offers to help him find his own way and get back on his feet. Soon after his interactions with Socrates, Dan begins experiencing different states of reality. Life literally slows down, and time stops, making it easier for him to start to see the beauty he's been missing out on, the subtleties of life.

Dan doesn't understand this right away and even thinks he might be going crazy, but as the movie progresses, he realizes that he's having an awakening of sorts. He's waking up to what's real, realizing he wasn't experiencing what was real before that.

I call this the crumbling. When what we perceive as our cornerstone of reality fades away right before our eyes, and then a new path or opportunity appears. Many of us have experienced this on a mass level in 2020. The crumbling of the reality we once knew. Only that old reality isn't going to work anymore if we want to grow and evolve. That's just how it works.

Your physical body is not you, and at the same time, it is important because it houses and directs your consciousness. It's fun to be in a physical body, and quite frankly, we must have one to exist in this reality. Without our bodies, there would be no point of reference for feeling and experiencing our lives.

That's why spiritual teachings are always suggesting not to over-identify with the body and to take good care of the body. While some people may take it too far and completely disconnect from the body, desiring a day when they can ascend into the ether, it's helpful to remember that your body is truly the temple that your consciousness is living in. Therefore, your body has to be in alignment for you to experience your spiritual potential.

I'm here to tell you there's a middle ground: not placing all your eggs in one basket with your physical identity, but instead valuing, appreciating, and loving your physical body. Taking the time to learn about all the subtleties of the physical and energetic body and how they interplay.

I've loved being in a physical body from the day I was born. If you'd asked my dad what I looked like right after I was born, he'd tell you I was born with my eyes wide open, curious about my surroundings. I was born curious and very excited to be here. Although I'm an adult now, this is still the energy I bring to the table.

ACTION STEP

What energy are you bringing to the table? At your very essence, how do you feel? Your best bet is to go back to childhood and remember the first feeling you had when everything was new to you. That's the feeling you carry on and want to rekindle into your adulthood.

CHAPTER 55

FROM HELPLESSNESS TO CONFIDENCE

LEARNED HELPLESSNESS IS A CONDITION THAT ARISES AFTER A person experiences a traumatic event and chronic stress. It's a condition in which a person experiences powerlessness, a lack of confidence and decision-making, and persistent self-sabotage, sometimes leading to depression.

I experienced what learned helplessness felt like firsthand after a serious back injury. At the time, I had no idea this was even a condition, much less the level of mental debilitation that came with it. It felt like I was in one of those dreams where you want to get up and run, but you can't because you're weighed down.

I felt sad, isolated, afraid, and quite honestly, helpless. I felt like I'd never be able to do the things I used to do, much less even feel strong again.

It was strange to me because I'd never felt this level of hopeless-ness in my life until then. When it was happening, I didn't even know I was in it until I got out of it and started to feel more like myself again.

I could have probably chalked it up to the back injury and, with that, some emotional trauma I'd been going through a few years prior. It was just too much for me to hold, and I realized I was also very nutrient-deficient. When I'd get emotionally stressed, I didn't eat. I'd also skip meals when I was busy. It all created a perfect storm for what was to come.

One day, I just stopped working out. Even though I was still a practicing trainer, I had no motivation to train myself. I felt as if I was living in another body. I was fearful that if I lifted weights, I'd reinjure myself and find myself in bed for weeks with back spasms, in pain, and crying uncontrollably again.

Until one day, I realized that I needed to start nurturing myself with the right foods more often. At the time, I didn't know how important this was. Sure, I knew high-quality foods were good to eat, but I'd not yet grasped the concept of low energy and what effect that had on my body's connective tissue.

Because I was energy-deficient, my connective tissue started to become inflamed, and the actual structure of my connective tissue became less stable and more restrictive. You see, your body will direct energy to the places that need it first, like your organs, before it directs it to the connective tissue, like your fascia and skin, if you're in a low energy state.

Since then, I've also seen levels of this in the clients that come to me. It usually gets sparked after some kind of physical injury that puts them in a state of fear of reinjury or after pregnancy.

Things like injury and pregnancy take a lot of energy from the body. Chronic stress, whether it's emotional, mental, or physical, your body doesn't really know the difference.

Another issue people run into is not being able to see the light at the end of the tunnel, so to speak. When we have lost our ability to see progress in small steps, this becomes an obstacle and ultimately slows down progress. Sometimes this even keeps you in a negative feedback loop that can be experienced as "learned helplessness."

It's a sense of giving up on yourself without even trying because you have this preconceived notion of hopelessness. There could be a clear way out, but you just don't have the energy to see it. This was demonstrated in an experiment with rats where the rats who had been shocked didn't even try to escape; they just gave up and eventually drowned.[10]

One reason this could happen is that there's a nutrient deficiency and a chronic stressed state that eventually leads to a severe low energy state. Most people underestimate the power of a severe low energy state amid trendy diets like intermittent fasting and low carb eating.

---

10 Martin E. Seligman and Gwyneth Beagley, "Learned Helplessness in the Rat," Journal of Comparative and Physiological Psychology 88, no. 2 (1975): 534–41, https://doi.org/10.1037/h0076430.

When we're in a low energy state, we don't have enough energy reserves to regenerate and heal the body, and not much is being diverted to cognitive abilities. Therefore, we end up in a vicious cycle of going nowhere fast. We spin in a circle of hopelessness and despair, essentially giving up on ourselves because we don't have the energy to see the light.

If you find yourself here, I suggest learning how to first build your body back up. Begin to create a food foundation with delicious, nutritious foods—foods you enjoy eating—and then learn how to manage your blood sugar properly by eating more frequent, smaller meals.

You want to make sure to include one serving of carbohydrates, protein, and fat in every meal. This is important because each macronutrient is dependent on the other to absorb nutrients properly. This translates to more even blood sugar levels and calmer internal systems so that you can experience your external world with a healthy disposition.

I've also found that eating breakfast is underestimated. It's a big deal. Just think of it like this: You've essentially already fasted the night before while you slept for around eight hours. Then you wake up, and there's a need to break the fast. This is essential for most people to lower their cortisol and adrenaline levels and bring them down to a normal place. Otherwise, you slowly begin to lose your appetite and may even start to feel nauseated from the excessive production of serotonin in the gut.

If you find yourself here, I recommend slowly implementing food back in by eating something that's easy for you to digest first thing in the morning until you're eventually able to eat more food without nausea and have an appetite when you wake up. This makes a huge difference in your energy levels throughout the day. It'll set the tone for your day, so make time for breakfast.

Foods like oysters, liver, and broth are ideal for healing and replenishing as well as aiding the thyroid for more efficient energy production.

Good carbohydrates support a healthy metabolism by providing the body with energy that comes from CO_2 production. This is way easier on your body in the way of energy production as opposed to producing energy from just protein and fat. Contrary to popular belief, an already stressed body will do much better and have a much easier time healing the metabolism by training the body how to digest carbohydrates properly.

I recommend starting by cooking your root veggies and fruits like apples and pears to make them more easily digestible. Add healthy saturated fat to them and eat them with protein. Eat tropical fruits in the spring and summertime.

If you've been limiting your carbohydrates for some time now, bring your carbs back in very slowly and in smaller amounts until you are able to work in a full serving at every meal. Carbohydrates will support your metabolism in a more efficient way, providing you with enough energy to recover from your workouts.

Then you'll be able to learn how to exercise mindfully, in a way that will build your body back up with strength and stability rather than depleting it with random workouts that may not give you what you need. You'll soon feel the strength and stability within, and again, this translates to your external world more than you may know.

What you experience from the inside gets projected to your outside, and this is what you experience. If you're feeling helpless, you'll experience yourself in the world being helpless, but if you experience the feeling of strength and confidence, you'll experience yourself in the world as such.

When my clients get stronger and begin to feel more confident and capable, they aren't scared that if they pick up something heavy, their back will go out. I think this might be the difference between arrogance and confidence. Arrogance is about feeling better than other people because you lack self-worth from the inside. With confidence, you feel capable, not helpless. You gain the ability and the courage to step one foot in front of the other and make progress each day.

In my case, I was able to do just that, and gratefully, I've been able to guide countless clients to the same place. What a difference it made to approach life when my tank was full and my mind was optimistic.

I learned how to build energy to create structure in my body, which ultimately saved my back. If you don't have enough energy, your structure will slowly degenerate. This feels like instability and inflammation.

I began to train my mind to think more optimistically, focusing only on how I wanted to feel, and stopped comparing myself to what I used to be. For example, I was a gymnast twenty years ago, and I could do things I can't do anymore because I'm older. More importantly, I haven't been training my body to do gymnastics for years, yet my brain was trying to compare my body to that.

I would say, "I used to be in such amazing shape—now look at me." Since then, I've heard some of my clients say similar things about themselves in the gym. Looking to the past and comparing themselves to what they once were.

This was a form of self-sabotage. To make progress, we must look at where we are at that moment and go from there. This will allow you to celebrate your wins, big or small. Otherwise, you just stay in a perpetual cycle of despair.

I soon realized each time I'd compare myself to my younger self and the shape she was in, I'd be giving myself an impossible task. Not to mention, there's no reason for me to be doing gymnastics anymore. Been there, done that. It's time for something else.

You end up never making any progress trying to re-create your past fitness regimen because you no longer need to be doing the same things you were doing in your early twenties, and you're starting from a new zero point, especially if you're coming back from an injury. You are a different person with different wants and different needs.

Now let's match our mindset to the body we want to create by becoming aware of our new values as we grow.

ACTION STEPS

Start by noticing any limiting words like "can't," "won't," and "should" and switch them for phrases like "I get to," "I could," "what if," and "I am."

Next, notice any resistance that comes up within yourself around these words. Are you able to move past the resistance and surrender to what could be?

Think about your point of reference now. What are you needing?

CHAPTER 56

LIVING IN THE VIBRATION OF BLISS AND JOY

"We must be willing to let go of the life we planned so as to have the life that is waiting for us."

—Joseph Campbell

PHYSICAL ALIGNMENT IS A SPIRITUAL EXPERIENCE. IT GROUNDS you and allows energy to flow freely through your physical body, allowing you to feel and have a point to reference for polarity.

Joy and bliss are a byproduct of this. Enjoying life and having fun are the ultimate spiritual attunement. The energy of joy and bliss are two of the highest vibrations. It's funny because when I use the word fun with most people, they tend to dismiss it. They almost see it as a weakness or something that's a waste of time, even though fun is what we all truly crave.

I believe bliss is a spiritual experience, and you can't find this without first learning how to play, make mistakes, and have fun. But it's hard to experience bliss until you've learned how to surrender to what you cannot control. It's more fun to roll with life most times and, of course, control what you can but let go of what you cannot and hand that over to the Universe or your higher self.

Our joy lies in the idea that many times, life does not unfold the way we always expect or plan, but it does unfold the way that is right for each of us. Giving us exactly what we need without losing anything. Oftentimes, the result is even better than what we could have imagined because we opened ourselves up to infinite possibilities.

Embracing the unknown in your life is like watching a good movie and waiting for the next clue as to what could come next with curiosity and excitement. What you discover along the way in your life is important, and it all relates back to you being able to see the beauty and bringing awareness to the synchronicities.

Your life is your greatest work of art. We are all artists in that way, and you get to create your life any way you'd like. That's the fun part, and having fun, I believe, is a spiritual experience.

So 5D wellness is all about discovering the beauty in your own health journey. Appreciate it and create unlimited potential within your limitations.

A perfect example is a client I mentioned earlier. She has astounded me as she's been through so much physically but continues to see the beauty in her own journey.

My client is doing things she never thought were possible and quite frankly that other people told her were impossible. She didn't know this about herself until she explored it and took inspired action to experience it. She shows up to each session twice a week on time with an optimistic attitude, open to laughing and having fun, knowing that she can trust that I'll guide her to where she needs to go. She's open to what she'll discover.

She comes to each session with optimism and a sense of fun. She's always sharing with me what she's noticed this week as an improvement in her body and in her movement. She notices the subtle changes, and I've noticed them too.

She's making incredible progress because of her attitude and her ability to see the beauty in it. This is so important because when you can start to learn how to harness this energy, you can do anything and enjoy doing it. It's the most high-vibe spiritual act a person can do.

That's not to say she doesn't voice her fears from time to time, but that's what I'm there for, to help guide her back to a place of stability and trust. We work as a team to create awareness around her unlimited potential, and it's beautiful.

She inspires me to keep going and never give up on myself too. I never know what each person is willing to accomplish until they do; I only see their potential. The rest is up to you.

ACTION STEPS

Have fun! What sounds fun to you? Do that. Put it on your calendar like all your other important to-do items. Fun is important.

Embrace the unknown. Can you release the idea of how your life "should" unfold and allow it to be the glorious adventure that it is? Can you find the joy in whatever comes your way?

CHAPTER 57

THE ENERGY
OF LOVE
AND APPRECIATION

*"The appreciation that Source feels for you, never-endingly, will
wrap you in a warm blanket of worthiness if you will allow it."*

—Esther Hicks, Jerry Hicks

THE HIGHEST VIBRATION WE CAN EXPERIENCE IS LOVE AND
appreciation. The energy of love and appreciation is what allows
us and everything around us to grow and flourish. Love and
appreciation reveal how we see ourselves in others. Ultimately,
this is the "oneness" that many spiritual texts talk about.

To appreciate and to love is an act of doing. You are directing
energy toward that person, animal, plant, place, or thing, thus
changing the quality of the energy. This is the ultimate action

step and one that will bring you the greatest sense of calm, pleasure, and joy in your body. What you are becoming happens faster when you can bring this energy into the mix.

The practice of presence leads to pure love. Pure love is unconditional.

At some point in the process, you realize you arrive at what we've been striving for. You are becoming, and then you are what you have been becoming. You reach a point of "being" instead of "getting to." Acknowledging this is the next step so you can love and appreciate the fruits of your labor right now.

The truth is, there's no distance between where you want to go and where you are in your life right now. There is no bridge to gap. It's an illusion that there is, but this illusion is necessary so that you get to experience what you'd like to experience.

A person who has seen this truth within themself will teach you how to see it and connect with it within yourself. Ultimately, you are the one.

What comes with this is an inner calm and appreciation for life that is unstoppable. You begin to develop a deep appreciation for everyone's role in it. You begin to see the unique expression that everyone in your life has to offer, including yourself.

Who and what can you appreciate in your life right now? How can you express love and appreciation to yourself in a way that is unconditional?

Your life is your greatest work of art. We are all artists, and you get to create your life any way you like. That's the fun part, and I believe that having fun is a spiritual experience. Enjoy your body right now. Love your body right now. Get close to your body, your mind, and your spirit. Celebrate the magnificence that is you!

ACKNOWLEDGMENTS

To my two sons, Murphy and Wilson, who have taught me how to be a better parent to myself and what it means to have unconditional love. I'm truly blessed to have you both in my life. You both inspire me to be the best version of myself. I love you both so much.

To my husband, Liam, who always supports me in every crazy thing I want to do. Thank you for believing in me, loving me for me, and always making me laugh. You remind me to not take life so seriously and the value of play. I'm so lucky to have you in my life. I love you!

Thanks to my mom for introducing me to my creativity early on and for possessing so many self-help books. Your curiosity to learn more about yourself through self-development impacted me greatly to help myself and to inspire countless others to be their best selves.

To my dear friend and talented writer, Kelly Sue Milano. Thank you for your guidance in helping me format and put all these concepts together in my book. You are truly talented. Writing a book is a process, and you've taught me that I can do it. I'm so grateful for your skills and your whimsical coaching approach. You are amazing. I'm so happy you were there to support me in this process.

To my dear friend and talented healer, Rosanne Grace. You've played an integral part in guiding me to both learn about and heal my inner child wounds. The skills I've learned from you have helped me transcend so much that I was able to write a book about it and share my experience with others. What a gift! Thank you!

To my amazing coach, Hanna Bier. Thank you for teaching me how to fully take responsibility for myself on all levels. You have taught me practical skills for managing my energy body that are invaluable and have made a world of difference in my life. I never knew how much I was truly capable of until I met you. Thank you.

To my dear friend, Laurel Arica. You have taught me what it is to be a true artist. You always inspire me to embody beauty and share my gifts with the world. Thank you.

To my mentor and dear friend, Paul Chek. I am so grateful I stumbled upon your book years ago. The work you and I have done together helped to break apart the tough armor I'd put around myself for years in fear that I'd be seen for who I was. You inspired me to think outside the box of what fitness really means and beyond. Thank you.

Many thanks to Josh and Jeanne Rubin, who have been a tremendous influence on my personal health, my understanding of nutrition, and how I help my clients to this day. You are both a valuable resource for nutrition.

To my coach, John McMullin. I am so grateful I not only discovered your classes and your work but also got to connect with incredible people who I consider my soul tribe. Thank you for everything you showed me about myself before I realized it in me. You have been a wonderful reflection and a powerful teacher.

RECOMMENDED READING

Anti-Factory Farm Shopping Guide, by Eugene Trufkin

Buddhist Mandalas, by Von Galt

Folks, This Ain't Normal, by Joel Salatin

The Four Agreements, by Don Miguel Ruiz

From PMS to Menopause, by Dr. Ray Peat

How to Eat, Move and Be Healthy!, by Paul Chek

Hypothyroidism, by Dr. Broda Barnes

Move Your DNA, by Katy Bowman

The Oxygen Advantage, by Patrick McKeown

Sacred Cow, by Robb Wolf

Unlimited, by Hanna Bier

Way of the Peaceful Warrior, by Dan Millman

ABOUT THE AUTHOR

ALLISON PELOT is a dynamic fitness trainer and energy coach specializing in rapid, permanent change through corrective exercise, metabolic nutrition, and energetic alignment. She helps people feel strong, confident, and calm in their bodies for life-changing results—with practical, proven energy skills including mindfulness, reflection, and deep affirmations.

Through Allison's signature mix of humor, entertainment, and authenticity, her podcast, *Integrate Yourself,* has inspired thousands to approach their health and wellness in a whole new way. Tap into your creative expression, understand yourself, embrace your joy, and create the body and life you want, starting right now. Learn more at www.finallythrivingbook.com.